ECZEMA-FREE FOR LIFE

ECZEMA-FREE
FOR LIFE

Adnan Nasir, M.D.
and
Priscilla Burgess

HARPER

NEW YORK • LONDON • TORONTO • SYDNEY

HarperCollins books may be purchased for educational, business, or sales promotional use. For information please write: Special Markets Department, HarperCollins Publishers, Inc., 10 East 53rd Street, New York, NY 10022.

FIRST EDITION

Image on page 41 based on illustration furnished by Dr. Jocelyn Thein.

Designed by Mary Austin Speaker

Library of Congress Cataloging-in-Publication Data

Nasir, Adnan.

Eczema-free for life / Adnan Nasir, with Priscilla Burgess.

p cm.

Includes index.

ISBN 0-06-072224-X

1. Eczema—Popular works. I. Burgess, Priscilla. II. Title.

RL251.N37 2005

616.5'1—dc22

2004054228

10 11 12 WBC/RRD 10 9 8 7 6

This book contains advice and information relating to health care. It is not intended to replace medical advice and should be used to supplement rather than replace regular care by your doctor. It is recommended that you seek your physician's advice before embarking on any medical program or treatment. You should seek medical care promptly for any specific medical condition or problem your child may have. Under no circumstances should medication of any kind be administered to your child without first checking with your physician.

All efforts have been made to ensure the accuracy of the information contained in this book as of the date published. The authors and the publisher expressly disclaim responsibility for any adverse effects arising from the use or application of the information contained herein.

From Adnan:
For my mother, Dr. Shafqat Nasir
For my wife, Angela
For my patients with eczema, their loved ones,
and their families

From Priscilla:
To all who yearn to live eczema-free

Contents

List of Illustrations xv
Acknowledgments xvii
An Introduction to Eczema xxi

PART ONE—UNDERSTANDING ECZEMA 1

Chapter One: Diagnosing Eczema 3

Skin Signs and Symptoms 4
Other Signs 10
Systemic Indicators 11
Signs That Point to Eczema 12
Related Disorders 14

Chapter Two: Managing Your Care 17
Managing Your Expectations 18
Working with Your Doctor 19

Chapter Three: The Physiology of the Skin 22
The Epidermis 23
The Dermis 25
The Subcutis 25

Chapter Four: The Genetic Basis 27
Immune System 29

Chapter Five: The Itch-Scratch-Rash Cycle 35
Itch Physiology 38
Itch Triggers 38
Types of Itch 44
Scratching 46
Eczema Rash 49

PART TWO—ADULTS LIVING WITH ECZEMA 51

Chapter Six: Daily Skin Care Routine 53
Inspect Your Skin 54
Treating Dry Skin—Bathing and Moisturizing 55
Causes of Itching 61
Watching Out for Infections 66
Managing Flares 73

Chapter Seven: Daily Life 75
Diet 75
Sleep 76
Stress 77

Clothing 78
Cosmetics 80
Deodorants/Antiperspirants 81
Fingernails 81
Sports 82
Pets 83
Cars 84
Finally . . . 84

Chapter Eight: Eczema-Free Home 85
Exterior Environment 85
Interior Environment 91

Chapter Nine: Managing Adult Life 102
Eczema at Work 102
Insurance Coverage 110
Traveling with Eczema 115
Sexual Health 117

Chapter Ten: Managing Your Emotions 124
Conquer Negative Feelings 126
Using the Mind to Heal the Body 131
Your Family and Your Emotions 134

PART THREE—FOR PARENTS OF CHILDREN WITH ECZEMA 137

Chapter Eleven: Caring for Your Child 139

Eczema and Infants 140

Caring for Toddlers 142

Caring for Older Children 143

Suggestions for Helping Itchy Kids 146

School Issues 149

Helping Your Child to Sleep 151

Using Steroids 157

For You, the Parents 159

Chapter Twelve: Psychological Impact 161

Children with Eczema 162

Lowering the Itch Threshold 164

Teenagers 165

Parents 167

Siblings 172

Therapy 174

Home Stress Reductions 175

PART FOUR—TAKING CONTROL 177

Chapter Thirteen: Treatments for Eczema 179

Treatments Supported by Research 181

Promising Treatments 183

Treatments That Require More Research 185
Treatments with No Supporting Research 189
Summary 191

Chapter Fourteen: Future Therapies 192
Research in Preventive Treatments 193
Attacking the Symptoms 195
Cure 198

Glossary 199
Resources 221
Index 233

List of Illustrations

The Atopic Triad 15
Cross Section of the Skin 24
The Skin's Barrier in the Epidermis 26
Causes of Eczema 28
Organs of the Immune System 30
Cytokine Balance 33
Itch-Scratch-Infection (Rash) Cycle 36
Key Players That Aggravate Eczema 39
Key Players That Aggravate Eczema with Central Nervous System Involvement 40
Eczema Skin Progression: Uninvolved to Chronic 41
Adult and infant/child rashing 231

Acknowledgments

Dr. Adnan Nasir writes: I have many people to thank who made this book possible. First, and foremost, I'd like to thank my wife, Angela, for her patience, persistence, and encouragement in helping me see this project through to its completion. I would like to thank the many patients and families dealing with eczema who have shared their lives with me and entrusted me with their care. Every day, they teach me as much about the strength of the human spirit as they teach me about skin disease. Their grace and resilience often leave me speechless.

I am grateful to the staff at Wake Dermatology (Dr. H. Mendall Jordan, Dr. Anne Tuveson, Sharon, Jill, Rita, Vickie, Suzie, Julie, Betty, Dee, Súe, Cheryl), who make coming to the office a joy and who perform magic every day to accommodate patients and referring physicians. I would like to thank my many medical colleagues and staff at Wake Research Associates. They have helped me tremendously with my clinical research and are responsible for bringing many discoveries from the bench to the bedside. It is in no small way due to their efforts that better treatments will be available for eczema each year. Dr. Ella Grach has been the chief source of momentum behind our research efforts.

I would like to thank my mentors in Iowa City, Rochester,

London, Boston, and North Carolina, who have not just taught me how to be a good clinician and scientist, but imbued in me the tremendous sense of privilege and responsibility that comes with health care. Dr. Anthony Gaspari took a chance on me when I was in medical school. Our research collaboration, which began over a decade ago, continues to yield fruit. He has epitomized the highest qualities of compassionate medical care, mentorship, and dedicated scientific research. Without his guidance, my life would have taken a different direction entirely. Dr. Lowell Goldsmith sponsored my career decision and made it possible for me to conduct research with Dr. Gaspari. Drs. Robin Eady and Malcolm Greaves taught me to always treat the patient and not the disease.

I would like to thank my colleagues at Duke University and UNC Chapel Hill for sharing their thoughts, knowledge, and advice in the care of my most challenging patients. Special mention in helping me with this book goes to Drs. Neil Prose, Dean Morrell, Robert A. Briggaman, Ed O'Keefe, Daniel MacAuliffe, Jo-David Fine, Pamela Guest, David Rubenstein, Richard Antaya, Fred Ghali, Navjeet Sidhu-Malik, and Russell Hall. I would like to thank the members of the vibrant and active Triangle dermatology community for their enthusiasm, their dedication to continuing education, and their camaraderie.

I would like to thank notable experts in the field of atopic dermatitis from around the world who have answered my questions, volunteered advice, and guided me through some of the more challenging concepts that I struggled to explain in this book. For help in the management of eczema, I would like to thank Drs. John M. Hanifin, G. Rajka, Donald Y. M. Leung, Carsten Flohr, and Hywel Williams. For providing insight into the mechanisms behind the immune system in eczema, I would like to thank Drs. Giampiero Girolomoni, Stefania Seidenari, Johannes Ring, Saveria Pastore, A. Braae Olesen, and Hitoshi

Mizutani. For providing information on the barrier, I would like to thank Dr. Phillip W. Wertz. For providing data on the usefulness of an education program in ameliorating eczema, thanks go to Dr. Alain Taieb and Dr. Jean-François Stalder. Some information on fish oil supplements for the treatment of eczema was provided by Dr. Martin K. Kagi. Many facts regarding the treatment of eczema in children were provided and reviewed by Dr. G. Ugazio. Useful information on eczema and breast-feeding was supplied by Dr. I. Sokolovski. The mechanisms of itch were made clearer to me by Drs. Gil Yosipovitch, Albert Fleischer, Toshio Ebata, and Stephen Feldman. I would also like to thank the many students and residents whom I have had the privilege to work with side by side. They may not know it, but they are the real teachers, and I learn from them.

I would like to thank Ted Weinstein for his vision and courage in seeing the importance of this project and taking on the risk. He and Priscilla Burgess have done enough work on this book to become eczema experts in their own right. I would like to thank my editor, Nicholas Darrell, for his steady hand, his clear view of the goals, and his keen interest in this project. Ted, Priscilla, and Nick have sacrificed tireless hours of personal time to see me through each stage of the manuscript. It was Nick's unflagging enthusiasm for the manuscript that brought the rest of HarperCollins's team wholeheartedly on board.

I would like to thank the North Carolina Writers Association for creating the nation's most active community of writers of all stripes. Their support and encouragement have been a boon. I would like to thank my writing colleagues and friends, many of whom I met through Erica Berkeley's workshop in Chapel Hill. Their comments, love for the written word, and companionship have kept me going through particularly slow periods. Special mention goes to my good friend Gillam Hall.

Everyone just mentioned has, in one way or another, contributed to my understanding of eczema and to the manuscript. All have volunteered their time, expertise, and advice. Any strengths in the book are, by all rights, due to their unselfish assistance. However, the responsibility for the final content, including all errors and omissions, rests squarely with me.

• • •

Priscilla Burgess writes: Thanks to Ted and Adnan for the opportunity to write this book, to Nick Darrell for making it even better, and to Jessica Chin who made it perfect.

An Introduction to Eczema

It's the relentless itching that makes eczema such an uncomfortable disorder. In spite of this, atopic dermatitis is commonly called *eczema*, the name of its most visible sign, the rash. For as long as people have been scratching, eczema has been one of the main culprits. Over thousands of years, myriad myths about its cause have been passed from generation to generation. Now, for the first time, scientists know that eczema is the result of the abnormal development of some twenty genes responsible for controlling how the skin interacts with the environment. The skin, when functioning properly, acts as a barrier to irritants and infectious agents. But for those with eczema, the skin's barrier function fails, permitting irritants to pass through to underlying tissues. These irritants trigger an immune response, the itchy rash that characterizes eczema. This new understanding of eczema is the result of revolutionary research in immunology and molecular genetics, now finally available to the general public.

With the discovery of the underlying cause of eczema, new and more powerful treatments with fewer side effects are being developed. It's now possible to provide accurate guidance for self-care that alleviates the terrible itching and painful rash. We now know, for example, that it isn't necessary to avoid dairy products, because diet has no effect on eczema. Oatmeal baths, on the other hand, recommended by Egyptian physicians thousands of years ago, actually do relieve the itching.

In 1975, 10 percent of the populations of developed countries had eczema. Today, the figure is 20 percent and increasing steadily. In the United States alone, nearly 30 million people suffer with this disorder, including 20 million adults and 10 million children. Eczema is the most common reason to visit a dermatologist and the third most common reason children are taken to a pediatrician. In 1998, over $8 billion was spent in the United States treating eczema. To complicate things, it rarely appears alone. Up to 80 percent of those with eczema also have asthma or hay fever.

Eczema is not a disease or an allergy—it's a vulnerability. Not every person with the abnormal genes develops eczema. Scientists believe that the cleaner the environment a baby is born into, the greater the chance the baby will develop eczema. Lack of exposure to dirt and other irritants prevents an infant's immune system from developing normally. Because of this, eczema typically appears first in infancy. Some rashes disappear at adolescence, but since the cause is a complex immune abnormality, eczema may continue into adulthood and symptoms can pop up at any age.

For an eczema sufferer, the discomfort of itching interferes with every aspect of life. It interrupts sleep, ruins concentration, and intrudes in relationships. Constant scratching leads to a red, inflamed rash, which is not only unattractive, but can also lead to serious infections. Eczema makes life miserable for both the afflicted and his or her friends and family. For some sufferers, the itching is so intense that life becomes unbearable. In extreme cases, intolerable itching has led to suicide. Many thoughtless and cruel fallacies have haunted eczema sufferers for too many years. The beliefs that eczema is a psychiatric disorder, catching, caused by something you did to yourself, or the result of being dirty aren't true and have encouraged people to treat those with eczema scornfully.

Research has shown that the more eczema sufferers know about the disorder, the better control they have over their symptoms. Even though knowledge is the most powerful tool for managing eczema, there is little factual information available for patients and their families. This book provides the latest medical information about the cause, symptoms, and treatments of eczema for both adults and children. In addition, it offers guidance for home care and ways to cope with the psychological impact of the disorder. *Eczema-Free for Life* will give you new hope and, for the first time, put control of your symptoms into your hands.

PART ONE
Understanding Eczema

Chapter One

DIAGNOSING ECZEMA

Eczema isn't like strep throat, which is easy to diagnose with a lab test and simple to cure with an antibiotic. There's no test to prove beyond a doubt that you have or don't have it. Instead, the diagnosis of eczema is based upon a careful search for a cluster of signs and symptoms. The itchy rash is the main symptom, but it's not the only one.

As soon as I enter the examining room, I'm looking for evidence. I analyze the signs I observe and the symptoms my patients report to see if they add up to eczema. Evidence can be found anywhere on the body, so, like me, your doctor might want to examine your whole body, even though you've come in because of a problem in a specific area. Signs of eczema can also be found in the eyes, lymph nodes, and other parts of the body, so don't be surprised if your doctor looks beyond your rash. The extent of the examination will depend upon how certain your doctor is of the diagnosis. Typical cases are easy to recognize, while atypical cases may require careful clinical evaluation.

To diagnose eczema, I ask the following questions:

- Do you itch?
- Do you now have a rash characteristic of eczema? (see pages 231–232)
- Have you ever had the characteristic rash of eczema? If so, did your rash develop before you were two years old?
- Has your skin been generally dry in the last year?
- Has anyone in your immediate family had asthma, hay fever, or eczema?

If you answer "Yes" to two or more questions, you probably have eczema.

SKIN SIGNS AND SYMPTOMS

While most people associate eczema with a red, itchy rash, there are other signs and symptoms, some of which are obvious even when there's no rash. The rash comes and goes, but evidence of eczema is always present.

Itch

Itch is the one symptom that must be present for a diagnosis of eczema. Itch drives patients to scratch, which triggers other symptoms commonly seen on the skin: inflammation, scaling, lichenification, scratch marks, and crust.

Inflammation

The redness of an eczema rash is actually inflammation. Scratching itchy skin damages cells. When the body perceives this damage, it sends defenses in the form of additional blood, immune cells, and other helper cells to speed healing. Besides turning red from increased blood flow, inflamed areas are warm to the touch and often swollen.

The degree of redness doesn't necessarily correspond with the degree of itching. For example, a bright red area may itch only slightly, while a light pink patch may be severely itchy. The brightness of the color may also depend upon complexion. In those with very light skin, any level of redness will be immediately obvious. For those with dark skin, the only clue to inflammation may be increased warmth of the skin.

Normally, the skin is a very efficient organ and requires little blood, about 2 tablespoons per minute. In the average adult, the skin is one-eighth total body weight, yet requires only one fiftieth of total heart output. This is because skin is usually metabolically inactive and the outer layers get some oxygen from direct contact with the atmosphere. With severe enough inflammation, blood flow to the skin can increase many-fold, and even deprive the body of needed oxygen and nutrients.

The skin of those with eczema reacts to scratching differently from that of those who don't have it. For example, if I write a word on a patient's back with a retracted ballpoint pen, a few minutes later the writing appears as a raised, dark red area with a subtle white halo. This reaction is found only in patients with eczema.

Occasionally, inflammation can cause your skin to hurt when touched. If it's affecting the hands, it can prevent fingers from bending and straightening properly. If there is widespread inflammation, you could feel ill. Severe inflammation is serious and should be treated immediately by your doctor.

Scale (Hyperkeratosis)

The eczema rash is not only itchy and red, it also often looks scaly. Eczema speeds up the process of shedding and replacing dead cells. This results in more dead cells on the surface of the skin than can be naturally brushed away. In some cases, dead cells adhere to one another instead of shedding, piling up into thick mounds that crack and flake off.

Eczema scale takes several forms:

- It may be fine and white like powder. When rubbed, it balls up, leaving red skin underneath.
- It may not be evident until the skin is stretched or bent, as in around the mouth or joints.
- It may be cracked, giving the skin the appearance of a dried mud flat.
- Sometimes thin, transparent sheets peel off like dried rubber cement.
- Scale may be thin and crumbly around the eyes.
- Scale on the palms and soles tends to be thick and rigid, often interfering with movement.
- It may be thick and yellow and come off only in flakes or chips, I sometimes use this as a diagnostic clue, so don't be alarmed if your doctor scratches and picks at your skin while discouraging you from doing the same.

A person with eczema typically has dry skin, so if the skin isn't thoroughly moisturized, it's possible that scale will appear anywhere on the body regardless of itch or inflammation. Scaling typical of the eczema rash tends to develop where the skin is thin and sensitive, like the eyelids, neck, nipples, and the inside of elbows and backs of knees.

Lichenification

Skin that is constantly scratched or rubbed will eventually look thicker, darker, and rougher than normal skin. Thickened, or *lichenified,* areas range in size from a pinhead to a dinner plate, depending on the location and how often and how hard the area has been scratched. Like calluses, lichenification is an attempt by the body to protect itself. Lichenification takes weeks or months to develop; however, if the skin is left alone, it will eventually return to its normal condition. Lichenification is found wherever the hands can reach. It's rare to see it in the middle of the back between the shoulder blades. Often, lichenified skin is darker than the surrounding skin, ranging from callus yellow in light-skinned individuals to the color of dried blood in African Americans.

Altered Skin Color

Constant scratching affects melanocytes, the cells in your skin that produce melanin, the chemical that determines the color of your skin. In some people, the irritation causes melanocytes to release extra pigment, and in others, scratching suppresses its release. If the melanocytes release extra pigment, there will be a brown spot where a patch of eczema used to be. If the release of pigment is suppressed, the affected skin will be lighter. This takes weeks or months to develop but will eventually go away if the skin is left alone.

I use a special light called a Wood's lamp to distinguish this condition from vitiligo, which is a permanent loss of skin color. Dark and light patches can coexist. If you have chronic eczema, you can have multiple dark and light spots in various stages of healing.

Scratch Marks (Excoriation)

Persistent, long-term scratching is a sure sign of eczema. The message to scratch an itch is generated in a nerve bundle near the base of the spine. The message then travels to the brain, but it also triggers an automatic scratch response to the itch. This is why some people are unaware of scratching. One patient told me she didn't realize she was scratching until she noticed blood on her fingertips. Another denied scratching while I watched him do it.

Typical eczema scratches are found in linear rows in places people can easily reach. Scratching the same area repeatedly damages the skin, and the result is a rash or lichenification. Most people are aware that scratching damages their skin and makes their rash worse, so they try pencils, pens, and wooden back scratchers rather than fingernails.

The damage done by scratching is determined by

- length, smoothness, and strength of fingernails. Jagged, chewed nails inflict the worst damage.
- how hard and long you scratch.
- whether or not you are scratching where skin is thinnest.
- scratching wounds before they have healed.

Crust

Crust on the skin means significant scratching or infection has damaged the skin to the point that it's leaking serum. Serum is the liquid part of the blood that was sent to heal the inflammation caused by damaged skin cells. As the air dries the serum, it builds up into a crust or a scab. Because patients with eczema tend to have an increased incidence of bacteria on their skin, I will often send swabs of crust to a lab to check for infection.

Cracking (Fissuring)

The impaired barrier function means patients with eczema have leaky skin. Moisture escapes, and the skin dries and cracks. Cracks form where the skin is constantly bent and straightened, the same areas where you find eczema rashes. Constant movement not only keeps cracks from healing, but also pushes irritants deeper into the skin. Without treatment, cracking spreads to ever larger areas. Visible, deep cracks resembling paper cuts are typically found on hands and feet. They're quite tender and very slow to heal. Most cracks, however, are microscopic and cause itchiness or irritation.

Small Blisters (Vesicles)

Eczema comes from the Greek word meaning "to boil over," which is a vivid description of the appearance of the skin during an acute flare, when it's common for blisters to form. One type of eczema appears only as clusters of tiny, itchy blisters on the hands and feet. If the occurrence of the blisters is sudden or unusual, it may indicate an infection, so I sometimes send samples to the lab to be tested. No matter when or where the blisters appear, they are always very itchy. In rare cases, blisters may be as large as a silver dollar, which prompts me to check for infection or even an alternative diagnosis.

Nails

I see patients with eczema who have come in because of damaged nails, assuming they've got a nail fungus or a nutritional deficiency. They don't connect the nail problem with their eczema, but that's often what it is. Eczema can damage the nails so they become thick and rough, pitted, or ridged. They can become infected. Nails that are dry will crack and split, sometimes along lines parallel to the nail plate. The dryness can extend to the skin around the nails, making cuticles peel and scale.

Sebaceous Glands

The sebaceous glands, which produce oils that lubricate and protect skin, don't produce enough oil in patients with eczema. This means they tend to have dry skin, but it also means they usually don't have problems with acne. The pores in the face of eczema patients tend to be small, making the skin look very smooth. I check for damage from harsh facial cleansers, exfoliants, and abrasive scrubs. These products tear down the skin's barrier, which the underproducing sebaceous glands can't help replenish.

OTHER SIGNS

Geographic Tongue (Lingual Erythema Migrans)

Eczema is associated with red patches of the tongue that gradually change their borders and migrate to other parts of the tongue over weeks and months. Geographic tongue typically causes no trouble other than its appearance, although it may be sore occasionally. It does need to be distinguished from fungal infections of the tongue, especially in patients who have been treated with steroids and antibiotics.

Eyes

It's possible to recognize eczema just by looking into someone's eyes. Irritated, itchy, and frequently rubbed during flares, the eyelids thicken and redden. Over time, they become puffy and dark, as if a patient hasn't had enough sleep. These are called allergic shiners, and 60 percent of those with eczema have them.

With each flare, the eyelids swell, then return to normal when the flare ends. This results in loose, saggy tissue around the eyes. The lower eyelids develop exaggerated creases, called Denny-Morgan folds, which make even infants appear wizened.

On the inside, the eyeball and the inner surface of the lids is covered by the conjunctiva. This smooth, lubricated tissue ensures easy eye movement and blinking. Eczema can inflame the conjunctiva, making it feel as though there's something in the eye, and a rough, inflamed conjunctiva can actually damage the eyeball.

A less common sign of eczema found in the eyes, keratoconus, is a change in the shape of the cornea from a gentle dome to one that looks like a rounded dunce cap. It's believed to be caused by constant rubbing.

SYSTEMIC INDICATORS

While eczema is usually thought of as a disorder that affects only the skin, a serious, chronic case can affect the health of the body as a whole. If I see a patient with widespread eczema, I check all basic signs (such as blood pressure and temperature) for indications that the eczema has become a life-threatening condition.

Enlarged Lymph Glands (Lymphadenopathy)

Lymph nodes are the body's germ filters. Cells in the lymph nodes learn to recognize the foreign substances that trigger eczema flares. This defensive process causes the affected lymph nodes to increase in size and tenderness. Swollen lymph nodes are never a good thing. They're strong indicators that the body is trying to fight off disease or infection.

Malnutrition

Chronic, severe eczema demands more resources than the body can absorb from the food ingested. This is immediately obvious in children who are small for their age. When the eczema is treated, they rapidly regain weight and start growing, often at a faster than normal rate to catch up. Adults with chronic and severe eczema tend to experience weight loss and fatigue.

Shock (Hypotension)

This is a dangerous and rare consequence of severe, untreated, or complicated eczema. If there is a widespread rash, the bulk of the body's blood flow is directed to the inflamed skin. To maintain blood flow to vital organs, the heart has to pump very fast. Less-vital organs sacrifice their blood supply for the sake of others by clamping shut their blood vessels.

Different parts of the body can tolerate this for varying periods of time. Muscles and bone can last hours. The gut, kidneys, and liver last minutes. The brain's blood supply is vigorously defended. Ultimately, the heart fatigues and is unable to sustain adequate blood flow. Multiple organ failures occur. Capillaries leak and blood enters the tissues. Circulation collapses. This type of shock is the equivalent of bleeding to death from the inside. When patients exhibit these symptoms, I hospitalize them immediately.

SIGNS THAT POINT TO ECZEMA BUT AREN'T PART OF THE DISORDER

Hair Loss (Alopecia)

I look for hair loss in patients with eczema for two reasons: First, it indicates where they have been scratching or rubbing excessively; and second, I can help them restore their hair if I catch it early enough. By treating the itch, patients stop scratching and the hair has a chance to grow back.

Hair loss from scratching can occur anywhere on the body; however, it's most obvious on the head because that's the first thing we see. Careful examination often turns up other patches of hair loss. Some patients with eczema on their scalps scratch so vigorously that they remove tufts of hair, leaving bald patches. If these are not allowed to heal, infection and scarring can ensue, leading to permanent hair loss. Thinning of hair of the outside edges of the eyebrows from incessant rubbing (also called Hertoghe's sign) is a well-recognized feature of eczema.

Pallor

The skin of some patients with eczema tends to have a grayish hue, accompanied by cold hands. Pallor around the eyes or mouth is a strong indicator of eczema. We don't know what causes it, but we think that in eczema, the tone or strength of the muscles that constrict blood vessels is greater than in people without eczema. When this sign is present, it's an additional clue that the patient has eczema. However, when it's absent, it doesn't mean someone doesn't have eczema.

Gooseflesh (Keratosis Pilaris)

When I see gooseflesh on a patient or the patient's parents, I've got another clue that points to eczema. Gooseflesh is caused by dry plugs in hair follicles on the upper arms and thighs and sometimes on cheeks. Gooseflesh doesn't itch or exhibit any other symptoms, but it's a marker for eczema. There may be no family history of an itchy rash, but if parents have this sign, they probably carry the damaged genes that can trigger eczema in their children.

Exaggerated Palm Creases (Hyperlinearity)

Hyperlinear palms have no symptoms—they neither itch nor hurt—but they provide another indication that the patient may have eczema. Skin (especially palms) that hasn't been scratched appears dry and crisscrossed with lines, like a salt flat overrun with motorcycle tracks. These lines are more pronounced in cooler climates and where the water is hard.

Cysts (Milia)

These tiny cysts are the result of plugged sebaceous glands on the skin, particularly around the eyelids. They look like miniature Ping-Pong balls, each the size of the period at the end of this sentence. They can grow two or three times larger. While they are not part of eczema, they can be exacerbated and infected if a patient has eyelid eczema. If they seem to be causing problems, I'll suggest removing them.

RELATED DISORDERS

Eczema is one member of the *atopic triad:* eczema, asthma, and rhinitis. These three disorders run in families and often appear together. Their exact relationship hasn't been absolutely determined, but, scientists believe the three share common gene defects. When diagnosing eczema, I always ask if these disorders run in the patient's family. If so, I can expect to find eczema.

Asthma

Asthma is considered the respiratory version of eczema. It's believed to be based on the same genes combined with lack of exposure to germs and pollen. In the case of asthma, the baby's

THE ATOPIC TRIAD

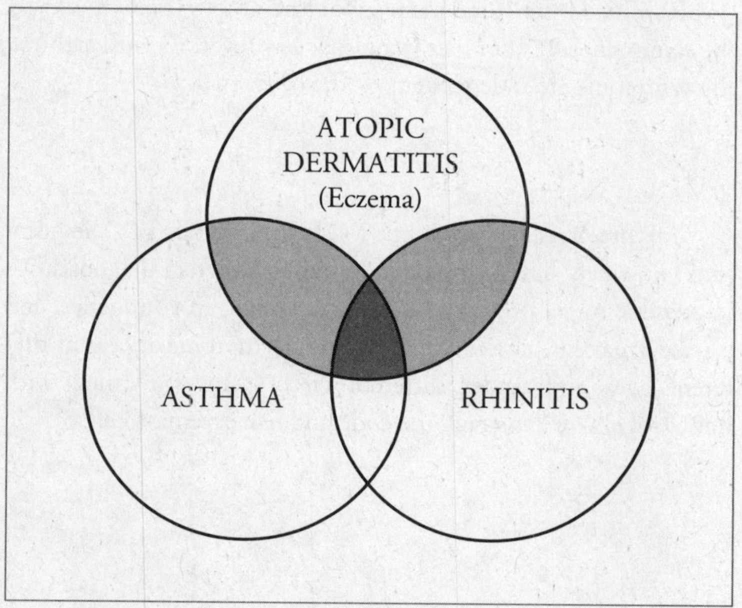

Atopic dermatitis or eczema overlaps with two other common disorders that make up the atopic triad. Subsets of people with eczema have either allergic rhinitis, asthma, or both. Furthermore, if a person has eczema, he or she may have a family history of any one or more of the diseases in the atopic triad. Some people with eczema don't recognize it runs in the family because they leave out relatives who have either just asthma or just allergic rhinitis.

respiratory immune system doesn't develop properly. It occurs in 10 to 20 percent of those with eczema. Typically, eczema appears first. If a baby's eczema is well controlled, it tends to reduce the baby's chance of developing asthma. If a person does develop both eczema and asthma, the two disorders appear to operate independently from each other. An eczema flare will have no impact on asthma, and an asthma attack has no effect on eczema.

Rhinitis

Rhinitis is the third member of the atopic triad caused by the same genes. It's familiar to most as hay fever. As with asthma, the symptoms are independent of the other two.

• • •

Eczema can't be cured, but it can be controlled to the point that you rarely have symptoms. Without a correct diagnosis, it's impossible to get proper treatment. Eczema is in your genes, and it's a permanent part of you. Different symptoms appear at different ages and under different circumstances. Armed with knowledge, you can crack the code and live eczema-free.

Chapter Two
MANAGING YOUR CARE

While your doctor is an important partner, you are the one who must be in charge of your care. To be eczema-free, educate yourself. Learn everything you can about the disorder. Research has shown that patients who have a solid understanding of their condition have a vastly better outcome than those who don't. Research is ongoing, so keep track of advances in treatments.

An educated patient combined with the right doctor is the formula for success. Dermatologists are the only doctors who specialize in disorders of the skin, but not all dermatologists specialize in eczema. You'll need not only a specialist for your long-term care, but someone you trust and like. Eczema treatment is a team effort, and you have to be as committed to managing your care as your doctor is to treating you.

Most people prefer doctors who provide patient-centered care. This means a doctor who takes the patient's quality of life and personal preferences under consideration in addition to medical issues. Your doctor should share information with you about the diagnosis, describe the full range of available treatments, and explain what you can expect from the treatments. For those with eczema on 100 percent of the body, treatment results can be dramatic. Treating those with small, itchy patches is actually more difficult because total eradication of symptoms sometimes just isn't possible.

MANAGING YOUR EXPECTATIONS

Eczema flares will occur no matter how carefully you take care of yourself. Sometimes treatments that have always worked before will fail.

The chronic nature of eczema can strain even the best patient-doctor relationship. Doctors are as interested in good results as their patients are. Eczema is a challenging and, at times, frustrating disease because it can be relatively slow to respond to treatment. When eczema does improve, it doesn't always disappear completely, and it frequently comes back. Victories are sometimes small and fleeting.

Don't limit your choices by jumping to conclusions or by thinking there are some treatments you'll never try. Talk to your doctor. Listen to what he or she has to say, then make up your mind. Because eczema is chronic, it's hard to continue to appreciate your doctor, but believe me, in the treatment of a chronic disease, a little appreciation goes a long way.

WORKING WITH YOUR DOCTOR

How Your Doctor Decides on Your Course of Treatment

Before prescribing a course of treatment for you, your doctor will take into consideration the following information:

- *Your age and sex.* Some treatments are not appropriate for some ages, nor would they be appropriate if you're pregnant or breast-feeding.
- *Your medical history.* Some treatments are eliminated because of other medical problems you had in the past. Be sure to tell your doctor what other medications you are currently taking to avoid harmful drug interactions.
- *The extent of the eczema.* Treatment will depend on the severity of the problem.
- *Your ability to pay for treatment.* Some treatments are costly, while others—such as a splash in the ocean—are free.
- *Your willingness to accept the risks of treatment.* All prescription medication has side effects, and some are worse than the condition being treated. A U.S. Department of Agriculture (USDA) study found that 96 percent of patients receiving new prescriptions didn't ask any questions about possible side effects.

Talking with Your Doctor

Many insurance companies require your primary care doctor to authorize access to a dermatologist. Insist on seeing a dermatologist who specializes in eczema, even if the primary care doctor offers to treat your eczema.

Many people find visits to doctors stressful. It's common to forget to ask questions or to discover that the answers have vanished from your mind as soon as you leave the examining room. If you need extra time to talk about treatment options, ask for it. Ask your doctor to go through your options step by step and write down his or her advice.

If your insurance company refuses to pay for eczema treatments, use the appeals and grievance procedures in your health care plan. Contact your employer's human resources department to find out how this is done, and ask for their help.

Questions to Ask About Suggested Treatments

Here is the kind of information you should know about any suggested treatment or medication. It's been organized into a checklist so you can easily go over it with your doctor:

- ☐ How long has this therapy been used for eczema?
- ☐ What are the potential benefits of the therapy?
- ☐ What are the potential risks?
- ☐ What percent of people improve on this therapy?
- ☐ How quickly will the therapy work?
- ☐ How long have you (the doctor) been prescribing this therapy?
- ☐ What are the most common side effects of the therapy?
- ☐ Will I be tested regularly for unwanted side effects? If so, what kinds of tests and how often?
- ☐ Which side effects will go away if I stop taking the medication? Which side effects might be permanent?
- ☐ Will I take or apply this drug continuously?
- ☐ Can I use/take this medicine for a short time, just to clear my eczema, then switch to a milder therapy with fewer risks? Could I control my eczema this way?

- ☐ Can this therapy be combined with another to decrease unwanted side effects?
- ☐ Can this therapy be stopped suddenly, or do I need to quit gradually?
- ☐ Ordinarily, how long will the drug stay effective?
- ☐ If it works but I have to stop using it, is it likely to work again if it is resumed?
- ☐ What will the therapy cost?
- ☐ If I decide against this therapy, what are my other options?

Once you and your doctor settle on a course of treatment, it is absolutely essential that you follow it exactly. Half of all patients for whom appropriate therapy is prescribed don't follow the treatment plan and, therefore, don't have successful outcomes.

Chapter Three

THE PHYSIOLOGY OF THE SKIN

Your skin is the barrier between your body and the outside world. It protects bones and organs. The skin regulates body temperature and fluid content. It provides protection from environmental assault such as ultraviolet radiation, microscopic organisms and irritants, blows, cuts, and scrapes.

The skin is the body's largest organ, weighing about ten pounds. It's made up of three main layers: the *epidermis,* the *dermis,* and *subcutis*. The epidermis is eczema's battleground. When a flare occurs, it's the epidermis that itches, flushes with inflammation, and looks rough after scratching. The dermis contains blood vessels, nerves, hair follicles, sweat and oil glands, and a multitude of other cells. The subcutaneous fat layer provides cushioning from impacts and contains major blood vessels.

THE EPIDERMIS

The epidermis is made up of several layers of cells (or *keratinocytes*) that start out as basal cells generated at the border with the dermis. Keratinocytes are shaped like rectangular cubes and contain primarily proteins and lipids. These cells are constantly being made, and as new ones appear, they push the older cells toward the surface of the skin, where they mature, die, and eventually slough off. This process takes about a month to complete in the young, twice that for older people.

As the cells are pushed up, they flatten and dry. Their contents spill out, creating a sort of mortar that cements dead cells into a strong waxy layer called the *cornified envelope*. The cornified envelope of those with eczema doesn't contain enough lipids to form a nice smooth layer or to moisturize the skin's surface. The epidermis dries out and cracks, breaking the barrier to the outside world. In addition, the dead skin doesn't slough off, taking with it germs and other irritants. Instead, the dead cells stick together, building up into a scaly pile where germs thrive.

Epidermal cells make antibacterial proteins called *magainins*. These proteins gather in pores and kill bacteria by punching holes in them. People with eczema don't have an adequate supply of magainins and are therefore more likely to be colonized by staphylococcal bacteria, which means constant staph infections.

The epidermis doesn't have blood vessels; however, it's alive with nerve endings that detect pain, heat, cold, and, of course, itch. Constant scratching in one area can lead to an increase in the number of itch nerve endings, making it even itchier.

The Basement Membrane

The *basement membrane* weaves the dermis and the epidermis together. The membrane has fingerlike projections that lock the

CROSS SECTION OF THE SKIN

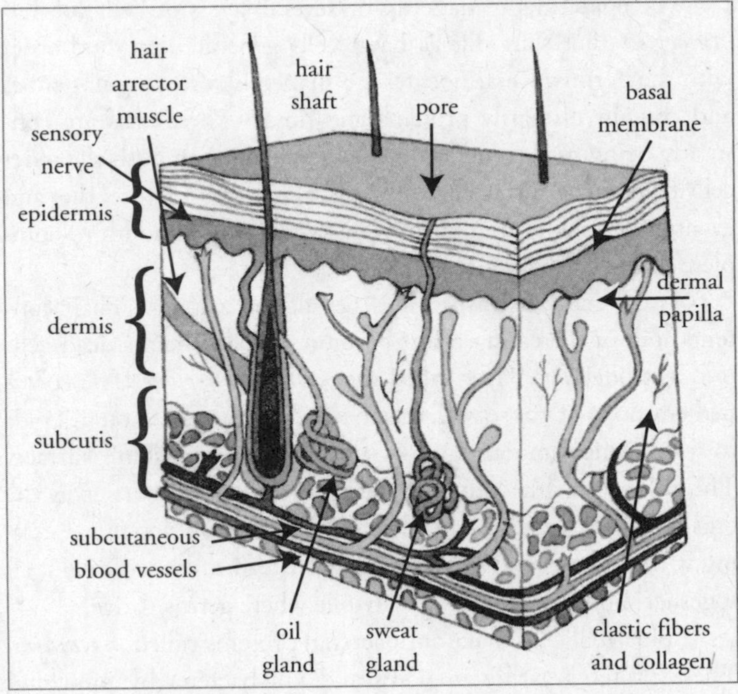

There are three principal layers of the skin. The *epidermis* is the outermost layer, and it is where the barrier resides (see 23). It is the first layer to contact the environment. The *dermis* lies just below the epidermis and contains blood vessels, lymphatic channels, collagen, and elastin. Lymphatic channels ferry foreign bodies entering the skin to lymph nodes, where they are filtered and neutralized. Blood vessels supply nutrients and are sources of inflammatory cells during eczema flares. Sweat glands originate in the dermis and empty out into the epidermis through small tubelike openings at the surface. Hair follicles originate deep into the dermis and penetrate the epidermis. Each hair follicle is attached to a muscle (which causes hairs to stand on end with fear or during shivering) and a sebaceous gland, which secrets sebum, an antibacterial and moisturizing oily substance. The *subcutis* contains fat and serves in shock absorption, thermal insulation, and calorie storage. Nerves can be found in all three layers of the skin and convey all types of sensation from pain to heat, to cold, to itch.

the two layers together like Legos. Each of the fingers, or *dermal papillae,* contains collagen, blood vessels, and nerve endings. This layer is sievelike, allowing free passage of various cells—blood and immune—to move freely between the epidermis and the dermis. Eczema doesn't exist below the basement membrane; however, if you scratch hard enough to draw blood, you've broken through the membrane into the dermis.

THE DERMIS

The dermis contains sweat glands that control body temperature. Sebaceous glands secrete oils that create the biofilm that gives skin its luster. This biofilm contains antibiotics that are deposited in the pores and kill off bacteria that might try to enter. While the dermis supports the epidermis, it actually has little role in eczema. Its main function is to provide the blood vessels that feed the epidermis and transport immune cells.

THE SUBCUTIS

Subcutaneous tissue contains sensory and motor nerves that detect touch. Fatty tissue is a shock absorber that also gives flexibility and resilience to the skin. This layer insulates the body from cold and the bones from trauma. Fat stores energy and nutrients, allowing you to live months without food. While important for the body, the fat layer has no role in eczema.

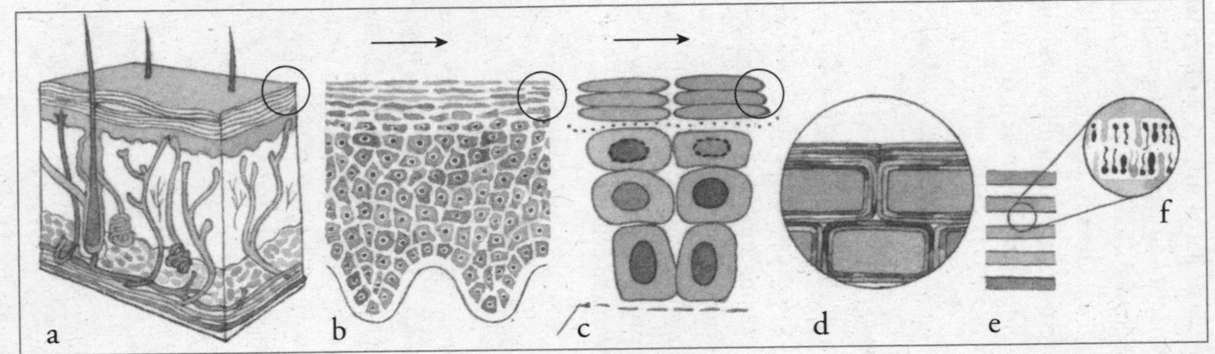

THE SKIN'S BARRIER IN
THE EPIDERMIS

The barrier has several components. The skin has a physical barrier and an immune barrier (see pages 40 and 41). In panel a, we can see a section of normal skin, with the epidermis, the dermis, and the subcutis. Panels b through f show magnifications of the outermost portions of the epidermis. Panels b and c show the overlap of cells in the epidermis, which resemble bricks stacked in a wall. These cells form a physical barrier because they are tightly woven together. They adhere to one another at many points and prevent the passage of substances around cells. Near the outer epidermis, the cells flatten (panel c) and develop hard outer envelopes (panel d) that are polymers of protein (panel e) and lipid (panel f). The polymer they form is analogous to Teflon. Like Teflon, these polymers are impermeable to the outside environment. They also hold moisture in the epidermis and keep it from drying out. In eczema, the barrier is weakened through microscopic cracks. Close inspection of the polymer in panel d shows it to be stacked layers of lipid and protein that is as hard and as impermeable as mortar, or grout between tiles.

Chapter Four

THE GENETIC BASIS

The inherited genes that create the potential for developing eczema are found on chromosomes 1, 3, 13, 15, 17, and 20. More may be discovered as the Human Genome Project continues. Normally, each gene functions as a set of instructions for a particular part or feature of our bodies. For example, a gene may encode eye color or the shape of the head. A single gene defect causes major changes, while multiple gene defects result in subtle effects.

As a multigene disorder, the type and severity of eczema differ from person to person. No two people (except for identical twins) will have an identical set of defective genes, nor will their bodies react identically to the environment. Often, eczema comes with asthma and rhinitis (hay fever) because there is an overlap in the genes responsible. Owing to the difficulty of identifying every gene involved in eczema, it's harder to analyze and measure than major single-gene defects.

CAUSES OF ECZEMA

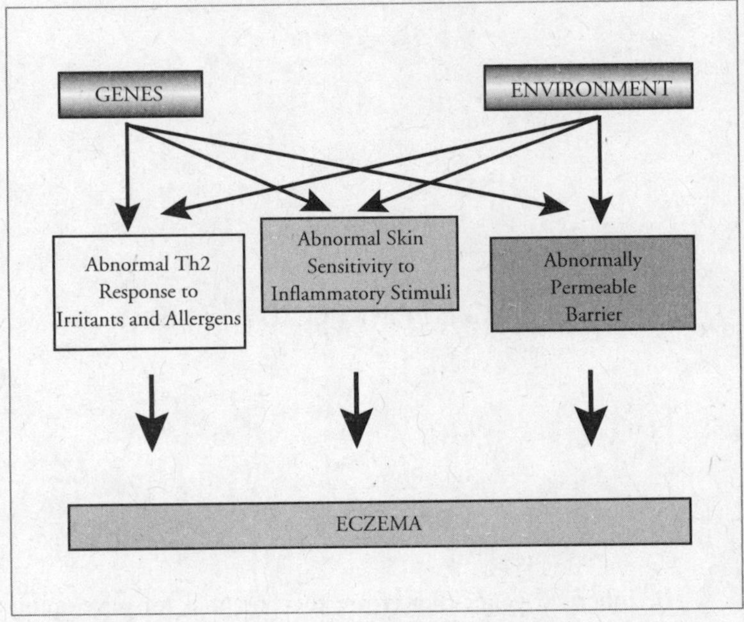

Multiple factors influence the development of eczema. Genes can compromise barrier function. They can make the immune system overreactive, or they can make the body respond abnormally to environmental stimuli. The environment can disrupt the barrier, or trigger the immune system. The bigger the environmental and genetic burden, the worse the eczema. Some individuals have multiple genetic and immune defects and in an unfavorable environment can develop severe whole-body eczema. Other individuals have only a few genetic or immune defects and if they live in a very favorable environment will have mild eczema or eczema limited to only a few small body areas.

We inherit half of our twenty-three chromosomes from our mother and the other half from our father. Together, they make up the full set of instructions from which our bodies are made. The instructions are encoded in DNA, which looks like a twisted ladder, called the *double helix*. There are four code molecules, abbreviated to A, T, C, and G. The number and order in which these four small molecules are connected to one another determine the makeup of each gene. Some genes are small, with only a few hundred letter codes. Others are made up of hundreds of thousands of letter codes.

The instructions encoded in the genes are sent via RNA, the genes' messenger, to the appropriate location. It carries the instructions, for example, for creating a perfect brown eye. If even one letter of the genetic code is missing or misplaced, or if the RNA gets its directions and instructions wrong, the results can be devastating. RNA is the template for proteins, which carry out the genetic instructions.

IMMUNE SYSTEM

The faulty genes responsible for eczema prevent the proper development of the skin's natural barrier and make the skin's immune function overresponsive. The leaky barrier allows more irritants to penetrate the skin, giving the already overresponsive immune system a never-ending supply of inflammation triggers. The immune system as a whole protects the entire body. However, some immune cells are given specific areas to patrol, such as the skin. Even though these cells have a defined area of responsibility, they are in constant communication with the rest of the immune system.

In addition to the chemical signals sent by immune cells, alarms are released by other kinds of skin cells. Epidermal cells, antigen-presenting cells, and mast cells in the dermis, the layer of skin under the epidermis, will send out an alert if they detect an invader. Antigen-presenting cells, like Langerhans cells, are always looking for invaders to capture. They dangle jellyfishlike tentacles in the middle and upper layers of the epidermis. If an invader gets caught, it gets taken to the nearest immune cell. If

ORGANS OF THE IMMUNE SYSTEM

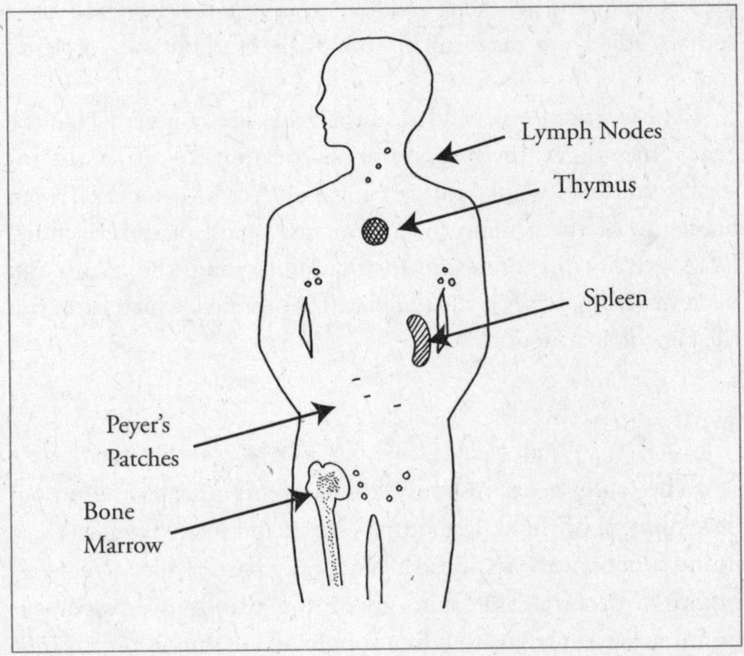

The immune system consists of organs and cells. Some organs manufacture cells (bone marrow), while others store them (lymph nodes, spleen). The cells do the work; the organ is where they reside or are made. Immune cells circulate constantly throughout the body. They patrol tissues via either blood vessels or lymphatic vessels. The organs of the immune system include the marrow of long bones (the source of all immune cells), the tonsils and adenoids in the back of the throat (which filter oral and respiratory germs), the thymus in the upper chest (where T cells are "educated"), the spleen in the left upper abdomen (which filters blood), the lymph nodes in the neck, the armpits, and the groin (which filter lymph), and Peyer's patches of the intestine (which filter germs in the gut).

the immune cell is nearby, the response begins immediately. If the immune cells are in the lymph node, it takes a bit longer. The chemical signals released by the antigen-presenting cells diffuse into the surrounding epidermis and dermis, calling for help.

These chemicals also trigger nerves to itch and blood vessels to dilate, to prepare for the impending rush of immune cells.

Immune cells are constantly communicating with one another. If the cells are in direct contact, they talk by sending signals to the other's surface receptors. If they're separated, they send chemical signals that float from one cell across to the other, where they're captured by a cell surface receptor that understands the message. When the other immune cells, regardless of their area of responsibility, detect the alarm, they rush to the skin's aid. In eczema, the emergency call for help usually triggers an overwhelming response to a false alarm.

Patrolling the Skin

The skin's immune cells travel in blood vessels to the capillaries of the dermal-epidermal junction, where they squeeze through tiny openings in the walls of the vessels. Now free to move around the epidermis, they search for foreign invaders. If none are found, they head back to the dermis and enter a lymphatic vessel for a ride to the lymph node. From the node, they return to the bloodstream to continue their patrol.

When Danger Strikes

In eczema, inflammation starts in the epidermis because that's where the invader is. The invading army typically consists of millions of individual particles. Meanwhile, there are usually only a few immune cells on patrol at any given place, at any given time. Reinforcements are called for immediately and do the following:

- The immune cells at the site "eat" the invader.
- The immune cells release chemical weapons that kill both the invaders and surrounding good cells.
- The immune cells release a chemical marker to guide

other immune cells to the site of the battle and chemical messages that attract more immune cells to the area.

- A few immune cells will take a few invaders to the lymph node, where they show the bad guys to other immune cells. The immune cells that don't recognize the foreigner stand idly by, while the cells that do go, into action. These cells divide rapidly, and their numbers grow astronomically. Soon there are billions of soldiers rushing to the battlefield.

Inflammation

The battlefield is the area of inflammation. The cells send out a call for help, and millions of immune cells make antibodies to attack the invader. This is good if the invader is harmful, like polio. It's not good if the invader is ubiquitous and ordinarily harmless like pollen.

Blood vessels expand to allow more immune cells to reach the area. This is the redness you see on your skin. The additional cells that rush to capture the invader cause your skin to swell. The serum that leaks through the spaces in the vessel walls made by the immune cells pools into blisters. The cells' chemical signals trip nerves and cause them to itch. This is done directly when an immune cell signal floats across to a nerve in the epidermis. The nerve is activated, and an itch impulse is transmitted to the brain. It can also be done indirectly when an immune cell signal goes to another cell, which then releases a signal that tickles a nerve.

To kill the invader, immune cells release chemical weapons. If the immune response is targeted and contained, as it should be, there is minimal "collateral damage." In eczema, the immune response is indiscriminate, and both good cells and invaders are killed. If enough of these killer chemicals are released into your body, you'll develop a fever and you will feel ill. An elevated body temperature does two things:

CYTOKINE BALANCE

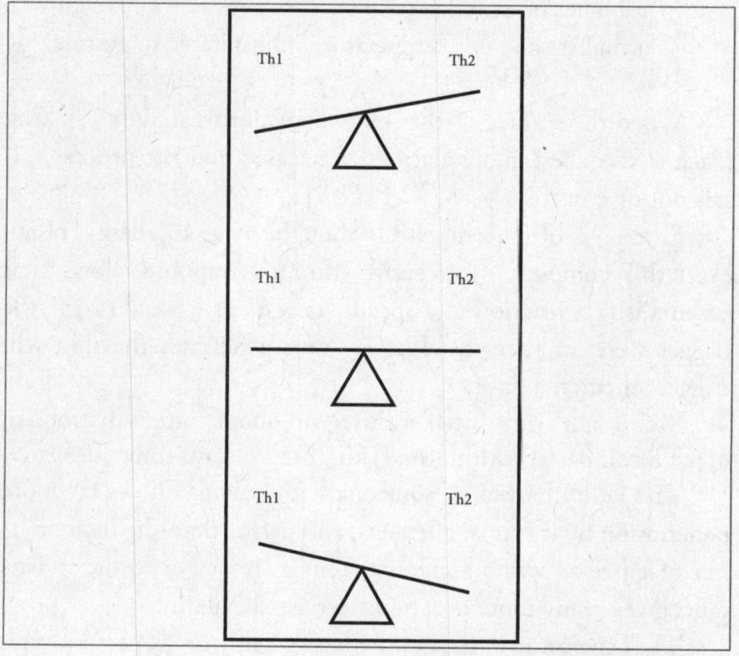

The immune system is normally fine-tuned. T cells are the quarterbacks of the immune system and call the shots when it comes to fighting foreign invaders. Different types of T cells have different roles and they carry out their roles by secreting chemical signals called *cytokines*. Different T cell types have different calling cards, or *cytokine signatures*. They also are useful in fighting different types of invaders. Two major varieties of T cells are Th1 and Th2. Normally, these are in balance. In eczema, there is an excess of Th2. Eczema treatments work either by suppressing the entire immune system (reducing Th1 and Th2) or by targeting the immune system more precisely (that is, boosting Th1 or selectively suppressing Th2). One interesting therapy for eczema is interferon, a known Th1 cytokine. This may work by boosting Th1 cells and restoring cytokine balance. There are other diseases—psoriasis, for example—in which Th1 predominates.

- It makes immune cells more efficient—they work better at higher body temperatures.
- It makes the body temperature inhospitable to germs.

When the surface of the skin where all this activity is taking place is scratched, more alarms are released and the process spirals out of control.

Eczema is often erroneously thought of as an allergy. However, this complex, overreactive immune response shows that eczema isn't a reaction to a specific trigger, as it would be if the trigger were an allergen. *Anything* that penetrates the skin will trigger an eczema flare.

We're not sure what's different about inflammation in eczema compared with normal skin, but we have some ideas:

The faulty barrier of someone with eczema allows far more penetration by irritants, allergens, and germs than the intact barrier of a person without eczema. This increased exposure to irritants gives many more occasions to raise the alarm.

The chemical messages between cells in a person with eczema are garbled. Some messages are interpreted incorrectly, and some are sent to the wrong place. It adds up to calling out a frantic false alarm that mobilizes an inappropriate immune response. The proper communication network of chemical messages among immune cells develops at, and shortly after, birth. If children are exposed to a full spectrum of germs at an early age, the immune system is balanced. If they live in a superclean environment, the immune system never has a chance to develop the correct communication channels. The Western obsession with cleanliness is most likely why the incidence of eczema is skyrocketing in the northern hemisphere.

Chapter Five

THE ITCH-SCRATCH-RASH CYCLE

Eczema is called the itch that rashes because it's the scratching that causes the skin to erupt into a rash. Many patients tell me that the itch is the worst part—they could put up with the red, flaky skin if only the itching would stop. Unfortunately, there isn't a test to evaluate how intensely your skin itches. Instead, doctors use a simple rating scale that ranges from 0, or no itching, to 10, which is the worst possible itch you can imagine. Doctors ask patients to select a number on the scale that they feel represents their level of discomfort.

The physiology of itch is the same for those with and without eczema; however, people with eczema have a heightened sensitivity to anything that causes itching. Where a gentle brush of a hand on a person without eczema will hardly be noticed, the same sensation for someone with eczema can trigger an itch attack.

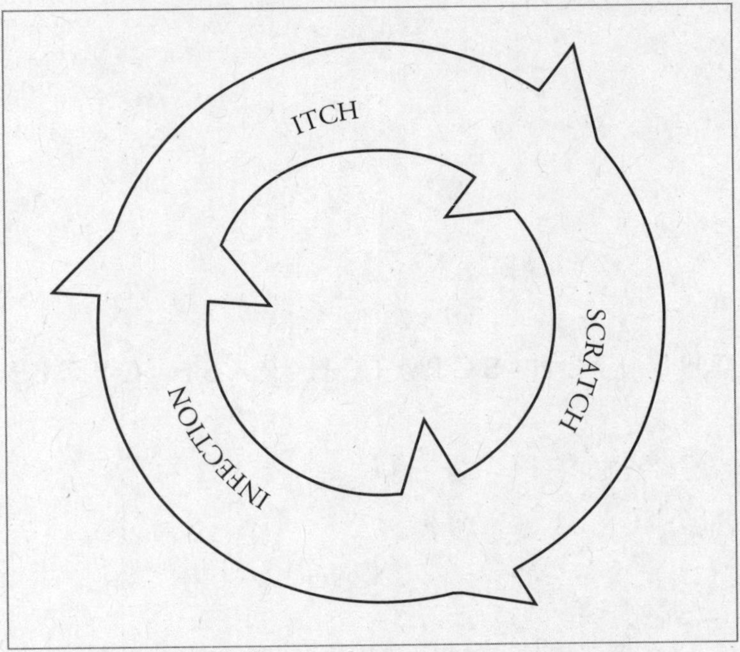

Eczema often spirals into a devastating itch-scratch cycle. Itching leads to scratching. Scratching disrupts the skin's barrier and makes it more vulnerable to irritants. These irritants cause more intense itching. Scratching triggers epidermal cells and cells in the skin immune system to release chemical signals. These signals cause itch. A scratched barrier is vulnerable to infection. Infection triggers the immune system to release even more itch and inflammation-inducing chemical signals. All of these itch signals lead to further scratching. While infection can take hours to days to set in, barrier disruption, irritant entry, and chemical signal release from scratching can take seconds.

Something that is only mildly itchy for someone without eczema will be perceived as intensely itchy for someone with eczema.

People with eczema also often misinterpret pain signals as itch. Inflammation can be painful to some, but in eczema, the same inflammation can feel itchy. This confusion of pain as itch probably resides in the brain. The brain is getting pain signals from nerves in the skin but is interpreting them as itch. Like pain, itch is a defensive signal that something potentially dangerous is on your skin. While pain triggers a rapid withdrawal, itch triggers the impulse to scratch out or brush away whatever is causing it.

It's believed that this reaction protects you from an insect bite, a parasite trying to burrow into your skin, or a plant or creature that releases dangerous chemicals. For those with eczema, this natural defense has gone haywire. Rather than alerting you that dangerous creatures or chemicals are on your skin, itching can merely indicate that a microscopic irritant has penetrated the skin's barrier.

While not definitive, there's interesting research that shows that some people with eczema have elevated levels of *immunoglobulin E* (*IgE*) in their blood. IgE defends the body against parasites. Scientists are exploring the possibility that the heightened immune response characteristic of eczema is the immune system trying to fight off a parasite invasion, even though there aren't any parasites on the skin.

There is no way to predict when the itching will start or how long it will last. Some episodes last for minutes and some can last for days, disrupting every aspect of life. Itch tends to be worse at night. Some think that when the mind is no longer occupied, focus shifts to the area that itches. Itching could also be triggered by too warm bedcovers, irritation from bedcover fabrics, and stress. One of the more promising areas of research is the effect of circadian cycles. Researchers have found that cortisol levels are highest in the morning and lowest during sleep. When cortisol levels are low, inflammation is high. Shifting the timing of treatment to match cortisol levels may help manage itching better, with less medication.

Many of my patients sleep poorly. Sleep deprivation leads to irritability, fatigue, and restless agitation. There have even been reports that for some, the only escape from the unrelenting torture of constant itching is suicide.

ITCH PHYSIOLOGY

The itch message is sent, via itch nerves or C fibers, to the *dorsal root ganglia (DRG),* a bundle of nerve cells near the spine. The DRG sends the message on to the spinal cord, where it is passed to nerves on the opposite side of the spine from where the sensation was first felt. This means that if your right arm itches, the left side of your brain will be alerted. These nerves carry the message to the thalamus.

The thalamus is a switching station for sensory signals, such as itch or pain. The thalamus sends the message on to the cerebral cortex, where the sensory cortex and the motor cortex are located. The sensory cortex is a map of the body that identifies the location of the sensation, in this case itch. The motor cortex and a scratch center deep in the brain stem trigger the scratch reflex so you can scratch the area that itches.

Unlike pain, itch nerve cells don't define a very specific spot. Itch nerves cover a fairly large area, up to 3 inches (85 millimeters) in diameter. The area is probably smaller on your hands and face but could be even greater on your legs. This makes finding the exact spot that itches difficult and causes skin that wasn't actually itching to get scratched as well.

ITCH TRIGGERS

For eczema sufferers, it seems as if everything in their environment triggers itching. To help you better deal with this very uncomfortable symptom, I'll explain what things actually cause

KEY PLAYERS THAT AGGRAVATE ECZEMA

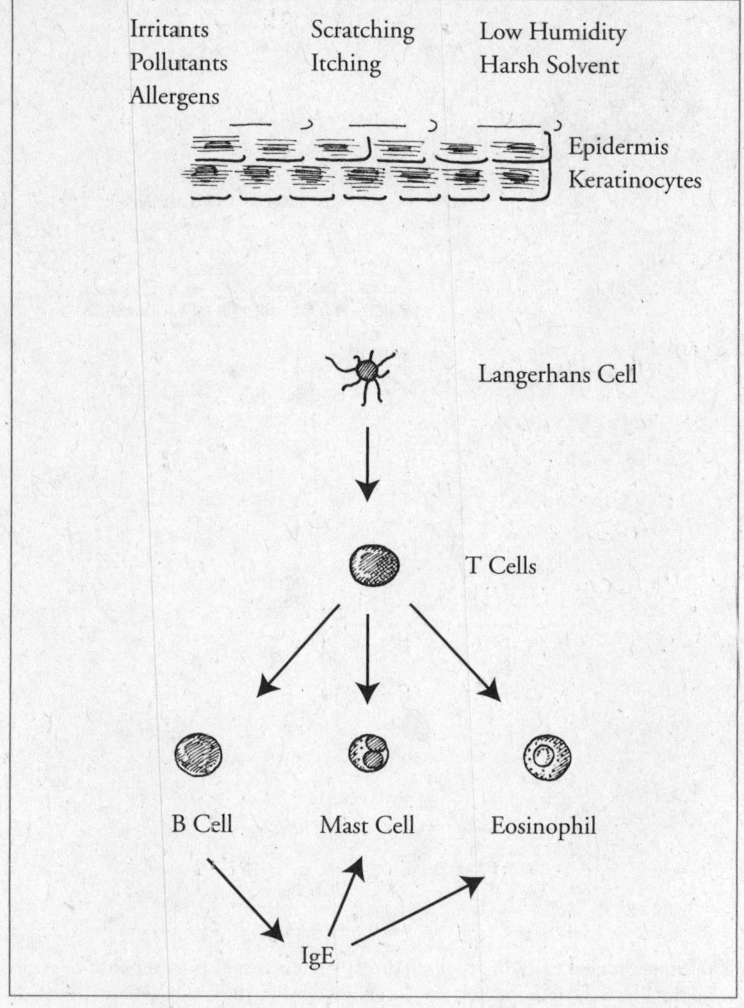

The epidermis in eczema is under constant attack from the environment. The skin's barrier is compromised in eczema to begin with, and environmental changes in humidity or decreased lipids or harsh solvents compromise the barrier further. It develops microscopic chinks, which allow irritants, pollutants, allergens, and germs easy entry into the epidermis and dermis. In the epidermis, these irritants encounter Langerhans cells, which present irritants/allergens to T cells. The T cells activate B cells to make the antibody IgE. IgE stimulates mast cells and eosinophils to release their contents, chemical cocktails rich in itch- and inflammation-inducing cytokines. T cells also directly activate eosinophils and mast cells.

KEY PLAYERS IN ECZEMA WITH CENTRAL NERVOUS SYSTEM INVOLVEMENT

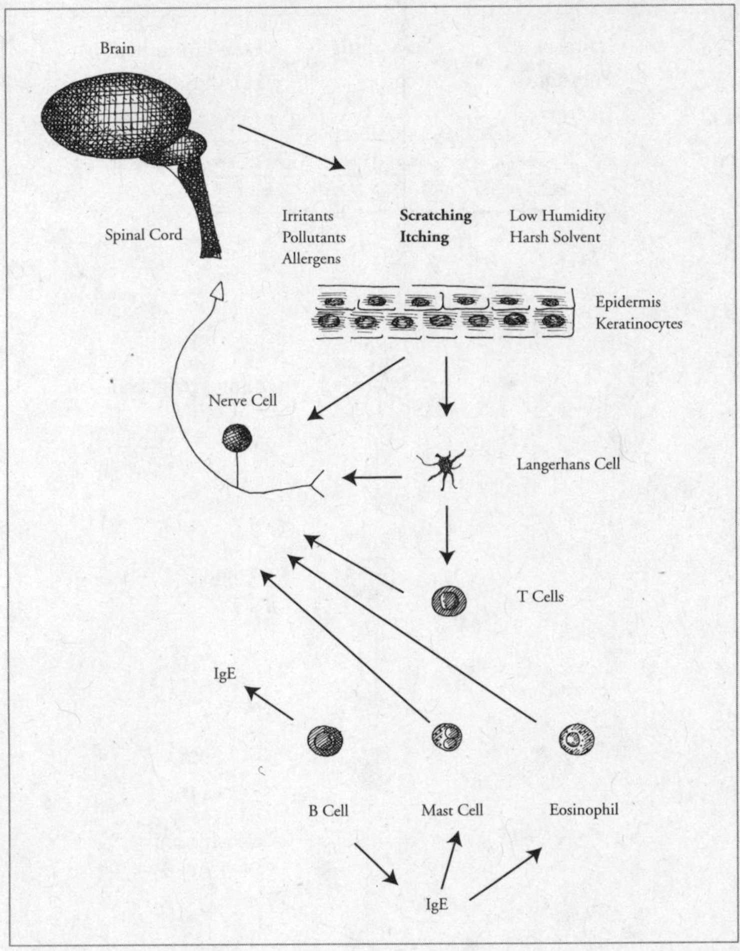

The supercharged cytokine cocktail directly triggers nerves in the skin to register itch. The itch signal travels up the spinal cord to the brain, where it induces the urge to scratch. Scratching occurs at the site of the cytokine cocktail. Scratching perpetuates the process in two ways. First, scratching epidermal cells causes them to directly release cytokines. Scratching also fractures the barrier, making it more vulnerable to irritants and allergens. Without the spinal cord (in paraplegia or, for example, with the application of a topical or injected anesthetic into the skin), there is no itch, and there is no eczema rash. Without the brain (for example, in deep, drug-induced sleep; or under the influence of sedating antihistamines; or in very young infants, who have not yet developed the brain enough to coordinate scratching), there is no itch, and there is no eczema rash.

ECZEMA SKIN PROGRESSION: UNINVOLVED TO CHRONIC

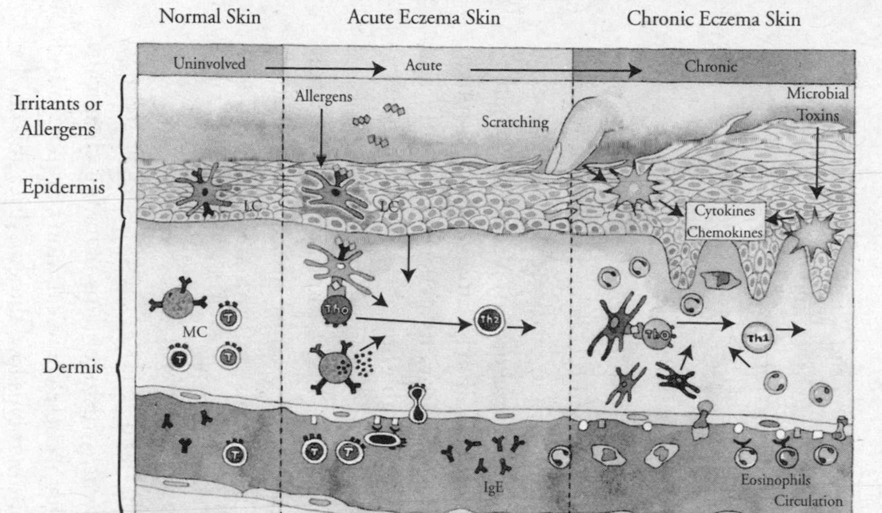

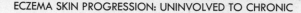

The left portion of the figure shows eczema skin before a flare. The epidermis is unharmed. Langerhans cells repose peacefully among cells in the epidermis. In the dermis, mast cells float unperturbed. T cells drift quietly among the collagen. Blood vessels have not unleashed their contents into the skin. The middle panel shows what happens when irritants enter the skin. They penetrate the weakened barrier and bind Langerhans cells. The Langerhans cells take the irritant to T cells and activate them to become Th2. The irritants also go to mast cells, and stimulate them to release their contents. These contents further stimulate a Th2 response. Cytokine chemicals accumulate in the dermis and make blood vessel flow increase; blood vessels also become leaky. More T cells, eosinophils, and antigen-presenting cells enter the skin. The cytokine cocktail induces itching and inflammation. Scratching directly triggers this process by damaging epidermal cells and causing them to release itch- and inflammation-inducing cytokines. On the right side, we see that the epidermis thickens. Blood vessels continue to leak, and the influx of immune cells becomes more dense.

itching so you can take the necessary steps to prevent them or at least keep them to a minimum.

Faulty Barrier Function

Breaks in the *stratum corneum,* the skin's surface, let irritants and allergens penetrate the skin. This would create an itchy sensation even without the additional itchiness triggered by an immune reaction.

Mechanical Irritants

Wool and fiberglass have tiny spines that can penetrate even a well-moisturized stratum corneum. These mechanical irritants trigger itching by puncturing cells or by directly pricking a nerve. Mechanical irritants lurk in unexpected places. Poor-quality makeup that hasn't been ground finely enough contains rough, spiky particles. These invisible irritants penetrate the skin and cause itching. Facial products with gritty abrasives can cause irritation, burning, and itching. Products made for sensitive skin are always best if you have eczema. Insect bites irritate by actually breaking the skin. Chemicals released by insects that penetrate the stratum corneum can also cause inflammation or infection.

Temperature and Humidity

Extremes in humidity and temperature can trigger itching. Hot weather triggers sweat, which contains irritating chemicals. When the humidity is high, these chemicals don't evaporate and can cause a flare. If the humidity is low, the skin dries and cracks, allowing irritants to penetrate.

Heat also expands the blood vessels in the skin. The body, including the itch reflex, works more efficiently when it's hot. At cooler temperatures, the body's chemical processes slow down, so itch isn't perceived as intensely. When it's cold, nerves that carry the cold message to the brain are activated. If you're cold enough, the cold message drowns out the itch message, so the brain perceives cold, not itch.

Irritants from Within

Stress hormones, alcohol, and caffeine make nerves more sensitive to itch. They work in different ways, but the end result is always itching.

- Stress hormones attract immune cells to blood vessel walls and help push them from the blood vessel into the skin. The immune cells then release *cytokines*, which work their way to itch nerves and trigger the itch message. Stress can also trigger the "fight or flight" response. In anticipation of pain, the body releases *endorphins,* which suppress pain but open the gateway to itch.
- Caffeine helps cells release *histamine,* a major itch trigger, and at the same time makes nerves jumpy. The combination of histamine and receptive itch nerves creates an intensified itch sensation.
- Alcohol makes blood vessels dilate, which increases blood flow to the skin. The temperature of the skin rises, increasing the skin's sensitivity to itch sensation.

Mind

There is no doubt that the mind plays a profound role in the perception of itch. Various techniques such as meditation, hypnosis, and even simple distraction can reduce the intensity of itching. On the other hand, focusing on itch can make it spiral out of control. Itch definitely has a physiological origin, but learning one of the aforementioned techniques can lessen its intensity.

No Obvious Reason

Sometimes skin itches even though you can't identify the trigger. It's possible that while carefully managing one cause, another may be lurking. For example, you might itch because of fiberglass that you weren't aware of. Or you may have reduced stress and controlled ambient temperature and humidity but forgotten about pollen or a pet that occasionally comes to the house.

Finally, not all itching is a symptom of eczema—it could be a symptom of a different disorder.

TYPES OF ITCH

There is no single cause of eczema itch, nor is there an itch specific to eczema. However, regardless of the type or cause, itching is always felt on the skin. Researchers have defined four types of itch, based on their causes. Unfortunately, it's possible to have more than one kind of itch at the same time.

Pruritoceptive Itch

This term means itching that originates on the skin. It's the most common type of itch experienced by eczema sufferers. It's affected by environmental factors like heat, humidity, stress, or medications, but it always begins in the skin. The imperfect skin barrier of eczema sufferers lets irritants and allergens penetrate the skin. The irritants by themselves are itchy, but for those with eczema, the immune system overreacts, triggering the release of chemicals that carry an even more intense message to itch receptors.

Other Types of Itch

These other types of itching are rare in eczema.

- *Neuropathic Itch.* This type is caused by a problem with the nerves that carry the itch message to the brain. Even though the origin of the itch is somewhere along the nerve, it's still felt on the skin. This kind of itch can happen to anyone, but for those with eczema, this type, combined with pruritoceptive itch, makes the itching more severe. An example of neuropathic itch is that experienced by people who've had an amputation and suffer from the "phantom limb sensation."
- *Neurogenic Itch.* While neuropathic itch is caused by disease along the nerves, neurogenic itch is a sign of a problem in the brain. It could be caused either by disease or by a drug that affects the brain. People with eczema who also have neurogenic itch can be tough to treat. That's why I like patients with eczema to know that in addition to their skin condition, they have to watch for other factors that influence itch. Opium-based pain medications, the antibiotic erythromycin, and aspirin can trigger neurogenic itch.
- *Psychogenic Itch.* True psychogenic itch, which is defined as the delusion of being infested with imaginary parasites, is rare in eczema. By definition, this type of itch has to occur in the absence of any disease. If you've got eczema, you've got a real reason to itch. Few individuals with eczema have psychogenic itch and need to be treated for the delusion as well as the real itch of eczema. These patients can elude accurate diagnosis for years. They switch dermatologists, making follow-up difficult. If I suggest they seek psychiatric care, they are offended since they don't think they have a psychiatric disorder. I have only a

handful of patients who fit into this category. Their lot is truly miserable, and they have to be handled very delicately. One unintended slight from me, and they'll disappear. Even though I don't have an itching disorder, I itch in the dermatology clinic when I see the intensity and fervor of patients' itching. That's also psychogenic itch. It's like psychogenic yawning—we yawn when others yawn. Eczema patients also can have this kind of psychogenic itch. They can be under stress, perceive itch, and deal with the stress by scratching.

SCRATCHING

If you itch, you'll scratch. There's no other way to stop the itching. Scratching is a reflex—you can scratch without engaging your brain. Some people are not even aware they itch until they realize they are scratching. Others who deny that they scratch will have marks on their skin, made while they sleep without being aware of what they're doing. The more you scratch, the more itch nerve receptors you'll have in that area. The release of nerve growth factors from damaged nerves makes the skin more sensitive to itch and more itchy for less reason. If scratched enough, itch trigger substances can become embedded in the nerves, causing persistent burning and itching. Scratching enhances the sensation of itching, creating an itch-scratch-itch cycle. An important part of eczema treatment is to control this destructive behavior.

Scratching makes itch worse in several ways:

- It physically damages the skin's barrier. This makes it easier for irritants and allergens to penetrate the skin and cause mischief leading to itch.

- It physically damages skin cells, which then release itch chemicals.
- It both damages itch nerves and tickles them directly.
- It pushes infectious agents into the skin. The infection triggers an immune response, which causes cytokines to be released, leading to itch.
- If you scratch long and hard enough, you'll damage the itch nerves to the point that they stop sending itch signals to the brain. Nerves can repair themselves in seconds, minutes, or hours, depending upon the extent of the damage. Once they're repaired, if itch signals are still present (cell damage, irritants, infection, or inflammation), itching resumes.
- Intense, vigorous scratching causes pain. Pain inhibits itch temporarily.

The nerve cells in your skin that send the itch signal to your brain are the same nerves that sense scratch.

How Scratching Works

There are several theories, but no absolute proof, about how scratching relieves itch. Here are some of the ways we think it works:

One Sensation at a Time

Your brain perceives one type of sensation at a time. If you itch, you won't feel pain or cold. If we assume that scratching is painful, then the brain registers pain, not itch. When the nerves that detect pain are activated in the same place where you itch, the itching can stop for hours. Some people with eczema prefer pain to itch. In a similar way, running mildly painful electric currents through itchy skin also relieves itching. It's also believed that the vibration sensation overwhelms the itch message.

Damaged Nerve Endings

Scratching may damage the nerve endings that carry itch to the brain. Fragile nerve filaments get bent or torn, which takes several hours for the body to repair. During this time, there's no itching.

Heat

The friction of scratching could raise the temperature of the surface of the skin to 110 degrees Fahrenheit, at which point itching stops. While mild heat can trigger itching, greater heat stops it. This is the reason hot showers feel so good to those with eczema. The problem is that very hot showers strip the skin's barrier and dry out the skin.

Rebuilding the Substance P Supply

Scratching tells cells to release Substance P, a chemical itch messenger that heads straight for itch nerves. When cells run out of Substance P, they start making more. While Substance P is being replenished, you don't feel itch. The nerve receptors that act on Substance P work most efficiently when the skin is warm but are suppressed when the skin is very hot.

Surround Inhibition

When an area of skin is scratched, nerve fibers around the site of the itch become numb and temporarily inhibited from working. It takes a while for them to perceive itch again. Researchers aren't sure why this happens but think it might be to sharpen the brain's perception of a new stimulus. So while the brain is focused on scratching, it doesn't pay as much attention to itching.

Scientists believe that these factors are active in eczema patients, but perhaps not all at once. This is why a simple solution often isn't enough, and getting comfortable requires a multipronged approach that involves preventing flares, treating inflammation, and blunting the effects of itch signals.

ECZEMA RASH

No matter how bad the itching, a person with eczema won't have a rash unless he or she scratches. The primary characteristic of an eczema rash is not how it looks, but how it feels: itchy.

The locations of rashes depend on the ability to reach and scratch an itchy area. In general, rashes develop on faces, necks, and in the bends of the elbows and knees. Eczema has several different rashes associated with it. The rashes depend upon the age of the person (see pages 231 and 232), the severity of the eczema, and complicating factors, such as infection. Acute rashes will be red, swollen, and crusty and sometimes develop blisters. In a subacute rash, you'll see redness on rough-textured skin. In a chronic rash, you'll see lichenification.

• • •

Eczema can be thought of as an itch-scratch-rash disorder. The skin itches, you scratch, and the scratching raises a rash. In my efforts to help patients, the ongoing focus is to prevent patients from itching so that this destructive and miserable cycle either doesn't get started or is stopped at the first sign of itch.

PART TWO

Adults Living with Eczema

Chapter Six

DAILY SKIN CARE ROUTINE

A consistent, medically sound skin care routine can keep most eczema under control. If you combine this with avoidance of environmental factors or circumstances that trigger your skin's immune reaction, you can also control the occurrence and severity of flares. Strict compliance to this routine will keep skin soft and clear of eczema for over 90 percent of those with eczema. However, many find it tempting, after an extended period of clear skin, to taper off the routine. Hot showers, perfumed soaps, and hasty moisturizing are sure to create havoc. Remember that your daily routine is absolutely essential for healthy skin.

This section describes a daily routine of bathing and moisturizing, during which you check for problem areas that itch, are infected, or are cut. I'll tell you how to take care of these problems. My goal is to help you create a world in which eczema is a background issue, not the focus of your life.

Schedule a time to examine and care for your skin. For mild eczema, this could take as little as 15 minutes in the morning and a few minutes at night. If you have total body eczema or a severe flare, it might take you 30 minutes twice a day. Once your eczema is under control, you'll be able to complete the self-care routine in just 15 minutes once a day. Careful attention in caring for your skin can keep you virtually rash- and flare-free.

INSPECT YOUR SKIN

Start each day with a good close look at your skin for areas of redness, cracking, excess dryness, and damage from scratching. Pay special attention to cracks—they allow irritants and infections to penetrate the surface of your skin.

- Look for areas of dryness.
- Identify itchy areas.
- Look for signs of skin infections like tiny pustules (pus-filled bumps), oozing or crusty areas, or crusty yellow blisters.
- Cuts and open wounds need to be watched carefully so that they don't turn into serious infections.

After you have identified problem areas, the next step is to treat them. The rest of this chapter tells you what to do when you find trouble spots.

TREATING DRY SKIN—BATHING AND MOISTURIZING

Proper bathing and moisturizing protects your skin by creating a barrier to the outside elements. This seems like a simple idea, but proper bathing is one of the most important steps to managing eczema, and many people don't know how it's done. Errors in bathing and moisturizing are *the* major cause of persistent eczema. There has been some confusion about the effect bathing has on eczema. Over the years, some experts have advised patients to stay out of the tub because water dries skin. Others have encouraged soaking to increase moisturizing.

Both perceptions are valid, but here's the solution to the confusion: Bathing will dry your skin if you allow the water your skin has absorbed while wet to evaporate. However, if you apply a moisturizer within 3 minutes of leaving your bath, the cream will seal in the water and create a barrier to irritants, keeping your skin soft and pliable. A patient who'd had eczema for years complained that no moisturizer helped her skin. I soon discovered that she waited until her skin was completely dry before applying it. She followed my suggestion to put on moisturizer within 3 minutes of leaving her bath and her eczema improved dramatically. If your skin is very dry or you're experiencing frequent flares, take 2 baths a day in lukewarm water, typically morning and evening. Here are some guidelines for effective bathing:

- Soak for at least 20 minutes—but no more than 30 minutes—until your skin (especially the tips of your fingers) wrinkles or prunes.
- Avoid washcloths, rubbing, scratching, and too much soap.
- If your skin is red and somewhat infected, add ¼ cup of chlorine (such as Clorox) to a tub of water. The chlorine will boost healing.

- If you like, add bath oil, but be sure to add it near the end of the bath when your skin is hydrated. Or you can apply it directly to your skin just before toweling.
- Bathing and shampooing just before bedtime will get rid of dust, dirt, pollen, and other irritants that accumulate on your body and in your hair during the day. This may help relieve some nighttime itching.

Oatmeal baths have been used by those with eczema for over four thousand years. This is one ancient remedy that is still recommended today. Oatmeal baths are very soothing, moisturizing, and healing. An added benefit is that they clean, too, so you don't have to use soap. Rather than stripping the skin of natural oils and acids like soap, oatmeal picks up dirt the way dough picks up flour. To make an oatmeal bath, put 2 cups of rolled oats in the blender, grind until fine, and add it to your bathwater. You can also buy prepared oatmeal baths (like Aveeno) at any pharmacy.

A brief, lukewarm shower is okay if your skin is under good control or if your flare is mild. Do your best to resist a long hot shower, even if you're symptom-free.

Soap

Normally, the surface of your skin is slightly acidic or, in other words, low on the pH scale. The acids in healthy skin protect it from infections and irritants. Those with eczema lack these acids. Most soaps sold in the United States have a high pH, which means they tend toward alkaline. Alkaline soaps, formulated to dissolve grease, wash away protective acids even on those with healthy skin, leaving the skin vulnerable to irritants.

Acidic soaps created specifically for eczema are sold in Europe and Asia, but none are sold in the United States. Dove has a neutral pH, neither acidic nor alkaline, and is currently the best choice available. Superfatted soaps, like Olay Sensitive Skin, leave a film of oil on the skin that gives the impression of moisturizing but actually contains detergents that dry skin.

Alternatives to Soap

You don't have to soap your entire body with every bath. Sometimes it's enough to rinse relatively clean areas with plain water, using soap only on areas that need to be freshened, like underarms, genitals, and the bottoms of your feet. Oatmeal is a good soap substitute. Here's how to prepare it:

- Put about 1 cup of rolled oats in the blender and grind until fine.
- Put the ground oats on a handkerchief and tie it tightly.
- Use it as you would a bar of soap.

Moisturizing

After bathing, gently pat off most of the water with your towel. Do *not* rub. Apply a moisturizer while your skin is still damp, within 3 minutes of leaving the tub and before you leave the bathroom. Apply a thin layer of moisturizer onto your entire body. Wait 2 or 3 minutes, then apply a second thin layer on problem areas. Two thin applications will be absorbed more easily and will coat your skin more completely than a single thick one.

About Moisturizers

There is a bewildering profusion of moisturizers to choose from, and not all are good for your skin. Most moisturizers contain alcohol, which is very drying and should never be used. Moisturizers should be free of artificial colors and perfumes. The newest and perhaps best moisturizer on the market today is Tri-Ceram cream. It contains ceramide, a natural oil found in healthy skin, and is available without prescription. Studies have shown good results when ceramide is replenished in the skin of those with eczema.

Moisturizers are distinguished primarily by consistency. Lotions like Vaseline Intensive Care Lotion can be poured, creams like Nivea are thicker, and ointments like petroleum jelly are the thickest. The thickest and greasiest ointments make the best protective barriers for your skin. However, most people don't want to go to work covered with petroleum jelly, so use the oiliest moisturizer you find acceptable for a particular part of your body. For example, you may not mind having a thick, greasy ointment on a patch of dry skin behind your knees but might prefer using a vanishing cream or lotion on your hands or face.

Use Your Judgment

There's much anecdotal information about adverse reactions to cosmetic ingredients and products, but few well-controlled scientific studies exist. This means that as a consumer, you have to pay attention to how your skin reacts to a particular product. Neither price nor brand name assures that a product will be of high quality or that it will not cause adverse reactions. Keep in mind that even the most inexpensive topical cosmetics are now tested thoroughly and screened to eliminate potential allergens, so the rate of adverse reactions to cosmetics and topical agents of most types is quite low.

Read the Labels: Ingredients and Terms to Look Out For

Some ingredients simply don't have an effect whether or not you have eczema. The molecules of the following ingredients are too large to penetrate the skin and therefore do not provide any benefit or consequence:

- RNA
- Protein
- Amino acids
- Collagen
- Elastin
- Nucleic acids
- Enzymes

Be careful about the term *hypoallergenic*. It means that all the ingredients are pure, but if you are allergic to the ingredient, it doesn't matter how pure or impure it is, you will develop a reaction. The terms *organic* and *all-natural* have very little medical meaning. Even among manufacturers, the terms have different meanings.

Many natural ingredients can cause allergies and irritation. The following *all-natural* ingredients have been known to cause a reaction in some people: allspice, almond extract, angelica, arnica, balm mint oil, balsam, basil, bergamot, cinnamon, citrus, clove, clover blossom, cocoa butter, coriander oil, cornstarch, cottonseed oil, fennel, fir needle, geranium oil, grapefruit, horsetail, lavender oil, lemon, lemon balm, lemongrass, lime, marjoram, oak bark, papaya, peppermint, rose, sage, thyme, wintergreen, and witch hazel.

Some synthetic ingredients are as good as, or better than, natural ones. For example, cyclomethicone, siloxane, and dimethicone are silicone-containing synthetic emollients that make excellent moisturizers.

Other compounds that claim to aid healing include jojoba oil, aloe, and vitamin E. There's no scientific evidence that these are helpful additives, but there is evidence that some people develop allergic sensitivities to these products.

Ingredients of skin preparations list chemicals that make it difficult to understand. These generally fall into five categories:

Emulsifying or dispersing agents are necessary when combining oil and water into a smooth, consistent mixture. Most are neutral and don't affect eczema. However, repeated applications of creams can cause emulsifiers to accumulate on your skin, which can lead to irritation. When patients use a cream that works initially, but then report that the cream is making their skin worse, I often suspect the emulsifiers. Emulsifiers include glyceryl monostearate, polyethylene glycol derivatives such as polyoxyl 40 stearate, or polysorbate 80. Sodium lauryl sulfate is an emulsifying agent that may irritate your skin.

Additives: The consistency and appearance of creams are improved by additives like cetyl palmitate and similar esters, which are neutral. Ethylenediamine is an additive that causes allergic reactions in some people.

Lubricants, emollients, and antifoaming agents include stearic acid, stearyl alcohol, isopropyl myristate, cetyl alcohol, or glycerin. These don't cause reactions in most people.

Suspending agents in pastes and ointments can include methylcellulose and gum tragacanth. These are both neutral.

Preservatives include parabens (short alkyl esters of parahydroxybenzoic acid), benzyl alcohol, oxyquinolone sulfate, organic quaternary ammonium compounds, hexachlorophene, parachlorometaxylenol, and chlorobutanol. These ingredients are neutral. Methyl- and propylparaben used as preservatives cause an allergic reaction in some people.

Years of problem-free use of a product is no guarantee that it won't irritate your skin in the future. Your body chemistry may change over time. Manufacturers reformulate brands with different ingredients so they can add "New" or "Improved" to the label. If you haven't had a bad reaction to your favorite moisturizer, keep using it. If you have acute or chronic eczema, you might want to see if a different moisturizer will improve the condition of your skin. If you are sensitive to many different products, trial and error, in combination with your individual preference, is the only rational way to choose a moisturizer. You may also want to see your dermatologist to get tested for skin allergies.

Choosing Your Moisturizer

When buying moisturizers, keep in mind the amount needed. It takes about 35 grams (about 1 ounce) of topical cream to cover the entire body. Typically, you need 10 percent less ointment than cream and 50 percent more lotion than cream. This is important to consider if you need to cover a large area, because costs can add up quickly, especially if you are treating yourself twice daily. Finally, it doesn't matter how appropriate a particular treatment is for your eczema, if you don't like it, you won't use it. If you don't like thick ointments, use a lighter moisturizer, even if it isn't as effective.

CAUSES OF ITCHING

Most studies show that in eczema, the itch comes first and scratching it causes the rash. In 1936, doctors performed an experiment to see if a little boy who was restrained from scratching would develop a rash. They covered his limbs and tied him down. The itching didn't go away, but when the bandages were removed, he had no rash. To keep the rash from breaking out, you need to control the itching. Treating itchy areas or areas that show evidence of unconscious nocturnal scratching should become part of your daily self-care routine.

According to reports by patients, the following are the most common itch triggers:

- Heat and perspiration, 96 percent
- Wool, 91 percent
- Emotional stress, 81 percent
- Vasodilatory foods (spicy foods like chili peppers or hot beverages like tea or coffee), 49 percent
- Alcohol, 44 percent
- Upper respiratory infection (cold), 36 percent
- Dust mite droppings, 35 percent

Many things can cause itching. Not every one will trigger itching in every person, but all of them have bothered someone with eczema. If you experience itching and can't figure out what caused it, take a look at the following triggers. You might find one you didn't know about.

Medications

Both prescription and over-the-counter medications have been known to trigger itching. If so, by law the manufacturer must report it in the literature insert that comes with all medications. *Be sure you read this information carefully.* Some medications that cause or worsen itch are opiate-based pain medications (such as codeine and morphine), antibiotics like erythromycin, or vitamin B complex.

One of my patients developed significant itching during her pregnancy. With her obstetrician's approval, I asked her to switch to a dye-free prenatal vitamin. The itching improved immediately. However, I don't know if it was the food coloring—many vitamins unfortunately contain dyes—or the B complex that caused the problem.

Idleness

When your hands and mind are free from other distractions, itching can become the focus of your attention. Some activities are so engrossing that you lose all sense of time and your surroundings. These can range from chess to archery to pool to bicycling to yoga. The key is to be engaged and active, not passive and idle.

Here are some suggestions:

- Keep your hands busy with squeeze balls, worry beads, or knitting.
- Play any sort of game: cards, Monopoly, or softball.
- Read a compelling book or magazine.
- Take part in an absorbing creative project, like writing, painting, or playing music.
- Watch TV.
- Cook, clean, or garden.

Nonchemical Ways to Soothe Itching

The desire to scratch can be overwhelming. Here are some ways to ease itching without damaging your skin:

- Apply firm, deep pressure (about equivalent to the weight of a bowling ball) to the site of itching for 1 minute. Apply the same deep pressure to the same place that itches on the opposite side of the body. Why this works is unclear, but the effect can last from minutes to hours.

- Try cornstarch. Cornstarch applied to itchy areas calms the itch. Don't put cornstarch in skin folds. Cornstarch contains glucose, which when combined with sweat promotes undesirable fungal growth.
- Use aspirin. Creams containing aspirin, like Aspercreme or Gold Bond Medicated Powder, relieve itch by inhibiting the chemical signals of inflammation.
- Use a cool tap-water compress for 10 to 15 minutes up to 4 times per day. This can be very soothing and relieve itch for hours. Here's how to do it:
    - Run cold tap water over a smooth cotton cloth. Wring out excess water.
    - Gently lay the damp cloth on the itchy area.
    - Keep it there for 10 to 15 minutes or until it loses its cooling power. Recool as needed.
    - When you have finished, apply moisturizer to lock in the water.
- Cold milk works even better because it has a higher cold-carrying capacity than water. For a milk compress:
    - Pour the milk into a bowl of ice cubes. Let it sit for a few minutes.
    - Dip a gauze pad into the milk, then gently squeeze out the extra liquid.
    - Put it on the itchy area for about 2 or 3 minutes or until it warms up.
    - Resoak and reapply for a total of 10 minutes up to 4 times a day.
    - Rinse your skin with clear water and immediately apply moisturizer.

Ice makes a good itch reliever, especially if the itchy area is small. Wrap a bag of frozen peas or corn in a soft cloth, then put it on the area that itches for 10 to 15 minutes. Wait 1 hour before you reapply the ice so you won't give yourself an ice burn.

Oral Medications for Itch

Taking oral antihistamines can reduce itching. They come in two varieties: sedating and nonsedating. Research doesn't show a clear benefit of antihistamines in controlling flares, but I have observed in many of my patients that they relieve itching. Sedating antihistamines have the added benefit of allowing you to get a good night's sleep.

While the packaging of sedating antihistamines warns you not to drive, drink alcohol, or operate heavy machinery, you should also avoid these activities with the nonsedating type, because in some people they cause drowsiness, especially in the elderly. Antihistamines will also make you less heat tolerant, so if you're planning to exercise, pay special attention to keeping cool.

Here are some of the sedating antihistamines on the market:

- diphenhydramine (such as Benadryl)
- chlorpheniramine (such as Chlor-Trimeton)

And one example of a nonsedating antihistamine:

- loratadine (such as Claritin)

Some antacids like Tagamet contain cimetidine, which is an antihistamine, so you get a double benefit: Both your skin and your stomach calm down.

Topical Medications for Itching

Pharmacies sell many topical creams for itchy skin. If you're using one for the first time, spread a bit of the cream on an unaffected area of your skin and leave it there for 24 hours to see if it causes irritation. If not, use it. If it does cause irritation, throw it away.

- Topical steroid creams containing 0.5 percent hydrocortisone are available without prescription. Use it once daily after your bath and *after* applying emollient to the skin. Apply only to the itchy areas.
- Topical aspirin can be used as an anti-inflammatory and itch reliever. Gold Bond Medicated Powder contains aspirin. *Warning:* Oral aspirin is not effective and may even worsen itch.
- Topical doxepin (Zonalon) cream may be applied 3 to 4 times per day.
- Calamine lotion is particularly good for cracked, wet, oozing skin.
- Lotions containing menthol and camphor (like calamine lotion or Vicks VapoRub) relieve itch by cooling the skin through evaporation.
- An application of local anesthetic gels with 0.5 to 2 percent lidocaine can soothe itching for about 4 hours. Use it 2 to 4 times a day.

WATCHING OUT FOR INFECTIONS

Although it may not be possible to avoid infection altogether, the seriousness of an infection can be minimized if it's identified and treated early. People with eczema and their families should learn to recognize signs of skin infections.

Cracks in your skin are portals for infection. If you have red, cracked areas covered with crust, try adding an antiseptic to your bathwater. I like adding Clorox bleach (¼ cup per full bathtub). In England, potassium permanganate 0.1 percent is used in bathwater as a disinfectant. Unfortunately, it leaves behind a permanent brown stain on your skin and your tub.

Topical Antiseptics

After your Clorox bath, you can apply a topical antiseptic on top of your moisturizer. Here are some you can buy without a prescription:

- Iodine (Betadine).
- Potassium permanganate, which is sold in aquarium supply stores as a fish tank cleaner. While it stains both your tub and your skin brown, it's a good alternative if you can't take antibiotics. It can be applied as a cold compress by adding ⅛ teaspoon to 1 gallon of water. Or you can add 1 to 2 ounces to your bath.
- Polysporin, a widely available, nonprescription topical antibiotic cream.
- Bacitracin (beware, as it is often found in combination with neomycin and polymyxin B).

Avoid products containing neomycin (such as Neosporin), which has been associated with allergic contact dermatitis.

Weeping Eczema

If your skin is oozing *(weeping eczema),* there are several different approaches to heal it. Try one at a time:

- Apply calamine lotion.
- Use a tap-water compress.

- For a saline compress, add 1 tablespoon of salt to 1 pint of tap water.
- For a vinegar soak, add 1 tablespoon white vinegar to 1 pint water.

When you're ready to use one of these treatments, gently clean the affected skin, then

- apply calamine lotion directly to the skin.

or

- dampen a clean washcloth in a lukewarm compress solution.
- apply to affected skin for 15 minutes twice daily.
- pat skin dry.
- apply moisturizer. Use a cream instead of an ointment if the skin is too wet.

Any one of these techniques dries cracked, oozing areas of skin, relieves itching, and heads off potential infections. Choose the method that feels best on your skin.

If you need to cover the infected area, use hypoallergenic Band-Aids or paper tape and gauze. The adhesive used on Band-Aids often causes skin irritation, even in those who don't suffer from eczema. Watch for signs that the infection is getting worse. If you see any of the following, call your dermatologist:

- The infected area becomes redder.
- Red streaks spread out from the site of the infection.
- It's painful to touch.
- The infection spreads to a wider area.

- The infected area drains yellow or green pus.
- You develop a fever (over 101 degrees F) or chills.
- You develop enlarged glands (lymph nodes) near the infection.

Insects

Insect bites require special attention if you have eczema. Research suggests you'll have a stronger reaction to insect toxins than those who don't have eczema. Start with the following techniques to reduce your insect appeal:

- Wear dark clothing.
- Cover as much skin as possible. Mosquitoes can detect unprotected skin the size of a dime.
- Wear insect repellent (try it out first to be sure it doesn't irritate your skin).
- Minimize time spent outdoors at dusk and dawn, when insects are feeding.
- Check yourself for insects and bites after being outdoors.
- Beware nights with a full moon. Many creatures are most active on these nights.

If you have a bite and you're sure it's nonpoisonous, here's what to do:

- Take an antihistamine like Benadryl.
- Put ice on the bite for 5 minutes. Repeat 2 to 4 times a day.
- Apply calamine or other lotion containing menthol or camphor.
- Alternatively, apply 1 percent hydrocortisone cream.

If the lesion doesn't get better or you think the bite may be poisonous, see a doctor. If you have a strong allergic reaction to insect bites (anaphylaxis), get a medical alert bracelet and ask your dermatologist about carrying self-injectable epinephrine.

Serious Infections

Failure to treat infected skin is the most common reason eczema doesn't improve after two weeks of consistent treatment. Some infections, particularly fungal infections, can mimic as well as complicate eczema. If you discover that you have symptoms of one of the following infections, see your dermatologist immediately. They can be cured only by prescription medications.

Staphylococcus aureus

This is the cause of 95 percent of all skin infections for those with eczema. Identifying characteristics are a red or yellow crust and yellow, fluid-filled pustules that may be painful or itchy. Staphylococcus can also cause boils or abscesses. Folliculitis is another staph infection in which pus-filled bumps appear around hair follicles in the hairy parts of the body. It resembles acne and in rare cases can cause the skin to shed in sheets. This is called *staphylococcal-scalded skin syndrome* and can be quite serious. If you suspect you have a staphylococcal infection, call your doctor immediately.

Herpes Simplex

Identifying characteristics are groups of water-filled blisters the size of a pinhead that tingle or hurt. This infection spreads quickly and can be serious enough to require hospitalization. Herpes occurs in a number of areas in the body. On the lips, it looks like a fever blister or cold sore. In the genital area, it looks like bubbling water blisters or open sores, usually with swollen glands in the groin. On fingers, it can look like a red, tender thickening of the digit, with or without water blisters.

Herpes is easily transmitted by skin-to-skin contact. It can be sexually transmitted or spread by contact sports like wrestling. Surgeons and dentists can get it from their patients, especially on their hands.

Once you have been diagnosed with herpes, be aware that you are infected for life and are at risk for recurrences at any time in the future. Learn to recognize your particular type of herpes and what your recurrence should look like. Call your doctor at the earliest sign of a herpes flare.

Candida

Candida is a yeast infection that can occur anywhere on your body. Most common for those with eczema are pus-filled dots in skin folds where the skin is beefy red. Candida also appears in other parts of the body:

- Corners of the mouth show cracking and scaling.
- Vaginal-area symptoms are itching and a cottage cheese–like discharge.
- Webbed spaces between the toes, where symptoms are skin cracks, pain, itching, and white discoloration of the skin.
- Fingernails, where the symptoms are thickening of the nails, white discoloration of the nail, redness, and tenderness of the finger around the nail.

Candida can be sexually transmitted to men from infected female partners. If you suspect you have this infection, call your doctor immediately.

Cuts and Scrapes

For those with eczema, minor cuts and scrapes have a greater chance of getting infected than for those without eczema. Any break in the surface of your skin, whether it's caused by a flare or a cut, makes infection easier to penetrate and spread. Infections also make eczema worse, so all cuts and scrapes must be tended to immediately to prevent complications.

Research has shown that eczema patients have a higher rate of *Staphylococcus aureus* colonization on their skin and in nasal passages than do those without eczema. The rate of colonization increases with the severity of dermatitis. This means that if you have eczema, your cut has a much greater chance of infection. Poor infection control and poor bandaging techniques prevent healing while making eczema worse.

Taking care of minor cuts and scrapes starts with stopping the bleeding and controlling infection. This promotes healing and preserves the function of the injured part. In the case of eczema, the goal is to prevent infection and preserve your skin. To control bleeding, apply pressure to the cut, preferably with a clean bandage or cloth. When the bleeding has stopped, clean the wound with lots of soapy water. Antiseptics won't help much if the injury hasn't been cleaned properly—in fact, antiseptics aren't necessary if cleaning is thorough. You might try benzalkonium chloride (Zephiran) or povidone-iodine (Betadine). Hydrogen peroxide is another good antiseptic. Petroleum jelly works just as well as any over-the-counter antibiotic dressing.

Bandaging technique is as important as cleaning the wound. A typical bandage consists of an inner layer attached directly to the wound and an outer protective layer that also limits movement to prevent reopening of the wound. Do not apply sticky adhesive to skin that is either injured or has a rash. If the injury is small and the skin around it is clear, cover it with a Band-Aid.

Larger wounds need to be covered with a dressing like petroleum jelly, a layer of absorbent gauze (this prevents contamination, absorbs drainage, keeps skin adjacent to the wound dry, applies pressure on the wound to limit bleeding, and protects the wound from further trauma), and an outer layer of either tape or a wrap to hold everything together and protect the wound from further trauma. If your injury is more than a minor cut or scrape, call your doctor or go to the nearest emergency room.

MANAGING FLARES

Flares happen. Sometimes there's an obvious trigger, like stress, contact with irritants, or infection, but most of the time they seem to come out of the blue. Small flares can turn into major flares if ignored, so be sure to take all necessary measures at the first sign. The first step is to be sure you're living an eczema-friendly life by doing the following:

- Check your home environment according to the suggestions in chapter 8.
- Maintain a cool, constant temperature and consistent humidity levels in your home or office.
- Limit your exposure to dust, cigarette smoke, pollens, and animal dander.
- Scrupulously maintain your daily self-care routine.
- Protect your skin from excessive moisture, irritants, and rough clothing.

- Prevent scratching or rubbing whenever possible.
- Look for infections or other complications.
- Assess your stress level.
- Get help immediately if you need it.

Meanwhile, take care of the flare by following a healthy self-care routine, taking oral antihistamines daily, and applying steroids according to your doctor's instructions. If your skin doesn't steadily improve to the point where the flare has vanished within 3 weeks, something else might be going on:

- Your flare was worse than you or your doctor initially anticipated.
- You or your doctor may have undertreated the flare, and you may need stronger medication and more aggressive care.
- There's an environmental trigger at home or at work that you may have overlooked. Check your medications, stress level, possible irritants, or allergens.
- You have an underlying infection.
- If you get better, but have a flare soon after (within 2 to 3 weeks), you may have relapsing eczema. In this case, you'll need ongoing treatment. To keep these patients clear, I have them perform self-care daily, then add medical treatments I've prescribed for weekends.
- Regardless of the reason, if you're not getting better, call your dermatologist.

Combining a good daily skin care routine with an eczema-friendly environment will keep your skin eczema-free more than 90 percent of the time. Following these steps helps you keep eczema from dominating your life.

Chapter Seven

DAILY LIFE

The next step in living an eczema-free life is knowing about personal habits and common products that can either make eczema worse or help it. Triggers lurk everywhere. Being able to identify them is a crucial weapon in the war against eczema symptoms.

DIET

I would like to emphasize that eczema is not an allergy, and it's not caused by food. A healthy diet that includes a wide range of food items is important for everyone. It's especially important for those with eczema, because having the disorder draws nutrients away from the rest of the body to feed the skin. Avoiding milk or following a restricted diet is not advised. However, if you have specific food allergies, such as peanuts, then you would of course avoid peanuts in all forms.

If you're overweight, consider losing a few pounds. Extra fat adds stress from skin rubbing against skin, and skin rubbing against clothing. Creases around the neck, under the breasts, in the abdomen, in the genital areas, and in the arms and legs can become irritated, infected, and a source of itching.

SLEEP

Getting a good night's sleep is important for everyone, but especially if you have eczema. Lack of adequate sleep, due to conscious or unconscious itching, or nocturnal restlessness is one of the major frustrations of the disorder.

At the turn of the last century, doctors recognized how badly eczema disrupted sleep. One of the treatments they used was to induce a "twilight sleep" with heavy sedation. Patients would sleep for twenty-three of twenty-four hours each day for up to two weeks. Their eczema and sense of well-being improved without any other intervention. Such a treatment would be impractical and unethical today, but it clearly illustrates the importance of sleep.

Recent studies show that patients with severe eczema sleep two and a half hours less than those without it. If you're not getting enough sleep, it will affect your mood, your sense of well-being, your relationships with your family, your performance at work, and your overall enjoyment of life. Here are some things you can do that might help:

- Adhere strictly to a daily self-care routine (see chapter 6).
- Avoid caffeine or other stimulants; these can cause itching and interfere with sleep.

- Allow at least 2 hours between your last meal and bedtime.
- Exercise regularly.
- Avoid daytime naps.
- Wear comfortable clothing to bed.
- For some, a bedtime ritual helps to relax:
  - Listen to soothing music;
  - Read a few pages of a relaxing book;
  - Self-massage;
  - Meditate.
- Sleep in a dark, quiet room.
- Keep the bedroom slightly cool.
- Stop itching by applying medication or lotion.
- As a last resort, take a sleep or relaxation medication.

STRESS

Although eczema is not caused by emotional factors or personality, it can be made worse by stress, anger, and frustration. Interpersonal problems or major life changes, such as divorce, job changes, or the death of a loved one, can make eczema worse or trigger a flare. Here are some suggestions that have helped people in difficult times:

- An informal support system of friends and family
- Eczema support groups
- Faith-based organizations
- Talk therapy, such as psychotherapy

In addition, here are some things you can do on your own:

- Regular exercise
- Meditation

- Relaxation techniques
- Yoga
- Massage
- Vacation
- Hire help to take care of stressful chores (cleaning, cooking, child care)

Consider occupational counseling if your job is a source of stress or if your job is unhealthy for your skin. In extreme cases, when you have to get away from a stressful home or a work environment that is making you sick, a "hospital holiday" can be prescribed by your doctor.

CLOTHING

In the past, clothing made only from cotton was recommended for those with eczema. However, research has shown that there's nothing special about cotton other than its smooth fibers. Silk and synthetics made with long, smooth filaments will be just as comfortable, as long as the cloth breathes. If the fabric doesn't breathe, your skin will get too hot, which might trigger itching. Wool and polyester have tiny, short fibers that prick and irritate skin. Regardless of fiber content, watch out for fabrics with a fuzzy surface.

Skintight clothing traps moisture and prevents your skin from breathing. Poorly fitted clothing rubs against your skin and can bring out a rash. Clothing labels can also irritate the skin, so you might consider removing them. Loose, comfortable clothing is always best. It's also a good idea to wear several layers of lightweight clothing, adding or shedding items until you're comfortable. This helps keep your body temperature under control. Rapid temperature changes can trigger itching, whether you're going from a warm house to a wintry sidewalk or from an air-conditioned building to scorching streets.

Laundry Products

Residue left by laundry detergents, fabric softeners, and anti-static products may aggravate itching. Running clothing through the rinse cycle twice gets rid of most of it. When washing clothing by hand, add 1 teaspoon of vinegar to each quart of rinse water.

Here are more tips:

- Wash clothing with enzyme-free laundry soap.
- Avoid detergents containing optical brighteners. Brighteners can cause irritation and itching without bringing on a rash.
- Dry cleaning doesn't make eczema worse. While dry-cleaning chemicals emit volatile organic compounds (VOCs), they have vanished by the time you pick up your clothes. Using "green" dry cleaners isn't necessary for eczema even if it's better for the environment.
- Avoid products with artificial colors and perfumes.

Protecting Your Hands—Gloves

The first line of defense for protecting your hands is gloves. However, if they aren't used properly, they can make things worse, especially for those with hand eczema. Wearing white cotton gloves is a good idea for routine activities that don't involve liquids. They'll protect you from irritants on the surface of things like newspapers and reduce friction on red, dry, cracked skin. Wearing gloves reduces the frequency of hand washing by keeping your hands free from grime. For situations where you need a good, strong grip, wear leather gloves or rubber gloves with cotton liners.

When doing wet work, don't wear latex gloves alone. They trap perspiration and moisture, which increases friction on your hands. Wear a dry cotton glove under the latex glove. If the cotton gloves get wet, change them for a dry pair. Consider using a scrub brush to wash dishes, and keep your hands out of soapy water altogether.

Be sure your arms above the gloves are also protected by long sleeves. When washing your hands in a public restroom, limit washing to your palms. They have thicker skin and can tolerate more frequent washing than the thin, easily dried skin of the backs of your hands. Hot-air blowers dry skin more than towels. If you have to use the blower, keep your hands at least 6 inches away from the machine, where the air is somewhat cooler. It's a good idea to carry something with you to dry your hands when you're away from home. Wear gloves when you wash your hair, or have it done in a salon.

The food you eat won't effect eczema, but the food you handle will. The juices of meat, vegetables (like potatoes, onions, tomatoes, and carrots), and fruits (like oranges, lemons, and grapefruit) are irritating and toxic to your skin. If you do a lot of cooking, be sure to wear gloves when preparing meals—or hire someone to help you.

COSMETICS

Use only hypoallergic cosmetics, like those manufactured by Almay. Check the list of ingredients and try to avoid products with preservatives, exfoliants, or irritants. Common ingredients to avoid are

- Benzoyl peroxide
- Alpha-hydroxy acid

- Glycolic acid
- Alcohol
- Retinol
- Salicylic acid

Stay away from harsh cleansers and makeup removers. For men, there are oatmeal-based shaving products, like those manufactured by Aveeno for Men.

DEODORANTS/ANTIPERSPIRANTS

Metallic salts in antiperspirants can irritate sensitive skin. If a deodorant contains any of these chemicals, don't buy it:

- Aluminum chloride
- Aluminum sulfate
- Zirconium chlorohydrate

Look for products containing the following nonirritating active ingredients:

- Allantoinate
- Zinc oxide
- Magnesium oxide
- Aluminum hydroxide
- Triethanolamine

FINGERNAILS

Artificial nails, applied at home or in a salon, can be a problem for those with eczema. Long, sharp nails do more damage when scratching; acrylics in artificial fingernails, sculptured nails, or nail extenders can irritate your eyes, nose, and fingers. Because we unconsciously touch our eyes throughout the day, we can rub irritants from the nails into our eyes. This can result in eyelid dermatitis. In some nail salons, bacteria or fungi exist in the equipment used, spreading infections from customer to customer. It's best to avoid artificial nails and to keep natural nails short and clean. Foot soaks in salons and spas have been associated with infections.

SPORTS

Extreme sweating and overheating can make eczema worse. For those who love sports, here's how to play hard and keep things under control. Pay attention to the things that can keep you cool and comfortable:

- Water always helps, both internally and externally: Drink it and mist your skin with it. However, excess sweat should be wiped away.
- Play in the shade, if possible.
- If there's no breeze, bring along a small fan.
- Avoid the midday heat by scheduling activities before 11:00 a.m. or after 3:00 p.m.
- If it's 90 degrees outside, you should probably choose a leisurely stroll around the golf course rather than a fast game of tennis.
- Wear comfortable clothing that is light in weight and color, topped off with a broad-brimmed hat or visor.
- If it's really hot, put ice cubes in your hat.
- Wear gloves for any activity that involves the rigorous use of your hands.

Eliminate as much friction on your skin as possible:

- Apply emollients between your thighs and on nipples.
- Wear smooth, slippery fabrics.
- Use powder to keep feet and underarms dry.
- Under padding, wear cotton clothing and a dusting of powder.
- Wear two pairs of socks, a thin, silky inner pair and a thick, cushiony cotton outer pair.

Take care of your skin:

- Swimmers need to rinse off and apply emollient immediately after a workout.
- Use sunscreens with labels that read "hypoallergenic," "PABA-free," or "dermatologist tested." Titanium- and zinc-based products are best.
- Check your opponent for a skin infection, especially if you're in a close contact sport like wrestling or synchronized swimming.
- Take cuts and scrapes seriously. Clean and bandage them immediately so that little scratches don't turn into serious infections.
- Use Ace bandages instead of adhesive tape, which can irritate your skin.
- Don't forget your lips. Apply lip balm with sunscreen.
- If lip balm is unavailable, periodically rub the side of your nose with your finger (it's rich in natural oils) and then rub your finger across your lips.

PETS

Unless you have a specific allergy to an animal, pets won't affect eczema, so don't get rid of them. The exception to this is guinea pigs. While the reason isn't known, their dander is especially irritating to eczema. Designating at least one room in the house a pet-free haven is probably a good idea.

CARS

Air-condition your car to keep out pollen, dust, and other irritants that may be harmful to your skin. If you react to pollutants while driving, you might want to check out cars that have built-in pollution filters. The filters recirculate air while you're driving through a particularly dense patch of pollen or pollution.

FINALLY . . .

It's possible that if you follow the suggestions in this chapter, you can keep your skin eczema-free and experience very few flares. The strongest prescription medications can't achieve what you can on your own. Understanding what irritates your skin and how to take care of it is the key to beautiful skin.

Chapter Eight

ECZEMA-FREE HOME

EXTERIOR ENVIRONMENT

Creating an eczema-friendly home starts with the actual building, its location and setting. This is especially helpful to keep in mind if you're planning to move or build. While it's important to keep eczema's enemies firmly in mind, don't forget its friends—plants that filter pollen out of the air and creatures that dine on pesky insects.

Site

In addition to considering schools, parks, and your commute, consider the things that aggravate eczema. Are there factories nearby? All factories release pollutants into the air—some more than others, but for especially sensitive skin, even a little is too much. Choose a neighborhood as far from factories as possible.

The dense auto exhaust that hovers over freeways and busy

roads creates its own pollutants, which also binds with pollen. This new pollutant is heavier, more irritating, and harder to wash off than either one on its own. It makes a miserable combination for those with eczema. You should avoid damp sites like those close to streams, rivers, or ponds. Low ground, like valleys, also tends to be damp even without streams or rivers nearby. High levels of moisture in your home encourage the growth of mold, dust mites, and other irritating particulate matter. If possible, choose a site that attracts fresh breezes, which will blow away pollution, pollen, and moisture.

Landscaping

The incidence of pollen reactions of all kinds has skyrocketed in the past fifty years. Those with allergies develop respiratory symptoms, and those with eczema experience inflamed skin. This increase coincides with a change in the kinds of plants gardeners choose. Where once male and female plants were found in equal numbers, today 99 percent of the plants in gardens are male. Female plants produce fruits and flowers that drop to the ground and create a "mess" that has to be cleaned up. Male plants simply release huge volumes of invisible pollen. This pollen was meant to be filtered out of the air by the flowers produced by female plants. Since female plants are rarely found near their male counterparts today, the pollen has nowhere to go and stays suspended in the air.

The first step to creating pollen-free landscaping is to be sure that male plants that release it into the air are either paired with female plants of the same species or not planted at all. A garden filled with female plants won't assault you with pollen and will sop up pollen from your neighbors' yards, too.

Increase the diversity of plants in your yard. Greater plant diversity will lead to greater diversity in insect and other wildlife populations, including pest predators. Some plants like marigolds and nasturtiums are naturally offensive to pests. Check with your local plant nursery or agricultural center to see what plants work as pest deterrents in your area.

Insects

Get rid of insects around your home. Drain any standing water that can be used by mosquitoes. To protect your skin from insecticides, look into chemical-free insect removers like outdoor bug zappers, adhesive gel traps like the Roach Motel, flypaper, or gas-powered military-quality carbon dioxide–generating mosquito traps. Mosquito Magnet and Mosquito Deleto are two brands available at Wal-Mart. Burn citronella lamps if you enjoy lingering on your patio at dusk. If none of these work, you might want to contact a pest control company to do a thorough job of getting rid of insects, especially if insecticides bother your skin. Keep in mind that insecticides will kill beneficial insects as well as pests, so before you start spraying, look out for the good guys:

- Ladybug beetles (feed on aphids)
- Dragonflies and damselflies (mosquito predators)
- Mosquito hawks (mosquitoes)
- Lacewings (feed on soft-bodied insects)
- Spiders (feed on any insect they can catch)

Bats, birds, frogs, and some fish can decimate insect populations. If you must have a pond in your garden, stock it with fish that eat insect larvae. Try not to step on your resident frogs, and do your best to keep your children from collecting them from your yard to stock terraria. Purple martins are one type of bird that eats mosquitoes. Check to see which birds in your area are the best insect removers, then put up the style of birdhouse they prefer.

Here are more things you can do to protect yourself:

- If you have a swimming pool, keep it covered when it's not being used and drain any standing water from the cover.
- A canopy of trees over your house will keep sunlight out and mold in.
- Bushes planted right next to the house will also encourage mold. Keep the bushes about 2 feet from the walls.
- Don't plant highly allergenic trees like birch, olive, pine, and privet.
- Cut the grass frequently to prevent it from flowering.

If you notice that your eczema gets worse after yardwork no matter how careful you are, leave the gardening to others.

Structure

Twentieth-century architects like Frank Lloyd Wright, Charles Édouard Jeanneret (Le Corbusier), I. M. Pei, Charles and Ray Eames, and Mies van der Rohe designed homes that would today be considered eczema-friendly. The lines are clean. The surfaces are easily dusted. The furniture is sparse, smooth, and accessible from all sides. Drapery and carpeting are kept to a minimum. Even the glass-and-steel boxy design of the buildings is eczema-friendly. The use of plastic and leather instead of fabric, laminates, and wood furniture denies dust mites a home and pollen a place to rest. If you're thinking of building or remodeling your home, a trip to the library for books about these architects' work is a good place to start looking for ideas.

Construction Materials

Many people think only of appearance when considering the materials used to build their homes. While looks matter, some of the attractive materials may contain dangerous chemicals. Other materials harbor uninvited guests like mold. Another major consideration is to watch out for dampness. Leaky basements or damp walls are not good if you have eczema.

A wooden exterior is the *least* desirable since it's more likely to harbor mold and pollen. Smooth, nonabsorbent surfaces are best. If you do use wood, get chemically treated timber to protect against dry rot and mold growth. Rot-treated lumber doesn't release synthetic VOCs and therefore won't trigger an eczema flare.

The preservatives and glues in construction materials emit gasses. Manufactured products like solvents, new carpets, aerosol products, and dry-cleaned fabrics emit VOCs. Invisible chemicals can penetrate your skin and cause irritation. To disperse these unwanted, invisible fumes, keep the windows open for the first few months you live in a newly constructed building if possible.

Check to see what kinds of materials have been used to insulate your home. Fiberglass insulation is especially harmful if you have eczema. The tiny fibers dig into your skin and are difficult to remove. Fiberglass insulation can cause severe itching, even in people without eczema. If you have eczema, stay away from attics and fiberglass insulation. Either have someone else in your family do the work or hire someone to do it.

There are alternatives to fiberglass, so if new insulation is in your future, consider one of the following:

- Blown or sprayed mineral fiber insulation is made from fiberglass, slag wool, or rock wool. Because blown fiberglass insulation is manufactured differently from fiberglass batting, none of the tiny particles that embed themselves in skin are released.

- Sprayed cellulose insulation is derived from organic sources like recycled paper products. This type of insulation doesn't release any irritating particles.
- Sprayed foam is injected into the wall or ceiling cavity, where it expands and solidifies. Foam doesn't contain particles that can irritate skin.

Fiberglass is used in many products in addition to insulation. I was surprised to see one of my patients return with a fiberglass eruption. I'd treated him after he'd cleaned out his attic and, at that time, told him to stay away from fiberglass. He swore he hadn't been in his attic for months, yet he was back with identical symptoms. After chatting for a while, he mentioned he'd been out in his boat, hit a rock, and had to patch the hole before he could get back to his berth. What was the boat made from? Fiberglass.

If possible, choose a home with a full basement so that the floor of every room has adequate air circulation to prevent the growth of mold and mites. Check your basement regularly for cracks in the foundation and leaks. Moistureproof your basement as often as necessary to keep it as dry as possible. Use your basement for storage only, never as part of your living space. When you do store things in your basement, make sure they don't become magnets for bugs and mold:

- Use moistureproof containers with moisture-absorbent packets like silica crystals or rice in salt.
- Keep out bugs by using cherry or cedar chests.
- Hang clothing in cedar- or cherry-lined closets.
- Put mothballs in stored clothing, but air or clean anything stored in them before wearing.

If you live in a tropical or subtropical climate, wash the exterior of your home periodically to remove mold, pollen, and dust. Clean your window and door screens with soap and water once a month.

Flooring

Floors need to breathe to stay healthy, so be sure there's some kind of buffer between a cement slab and your flooring. This is especially important if you have wall-to-wall carpets. Lack of air circulation and slow moisture evaporation creates dust mite heaven. Better yet, don't use wall-to-wall carpets at all. Polished wood (smooth, not grooved), tile, vinyl, linoleum, or marble are the best types of flooring for those with eczema. Ceramic tiles are best for bathrooms and kitchens. Avoid porous, unsealed tiles that can harbor bacteria and other microorganisms. If you do have porous tiles in your home, seal them.

INTERIOR ENVIRONMENT

If you can't control your exterior environment, you can take steps to manage the interior. Equipment like temperature and filtering systems will keep temperature, humidity, and airborne pollutants at comfortable levels. The ideal situation is to balance your indoor and outdoor environments, but if you can't, the following suggestions will provide comfort.

Temperature

Cool air has an anesthetic effect on skin and helps to minimize itching. If the air is too warm, the blood vessels in your skin dilate. This can cause a tingling or itchy sensation. Maintaining indoor temperatures at 65 degrees F (18 degrees centigrade) should keep you comfortable.

Heating

Even if it's really cold outside, keep the heat in your home at about 65 degrees F. Overheating is a major cause of eczema flares. Patients who have forced-air heating systems seem to report more flares in winter than those with other types of heating systems. Radiant heating is the ideal system for keeping warm without irritating your skin. Avoid gas heaters because they reduce humidity in the winter. Wood or coal fires do not aggravate eczema. If you're considering a wood-burning stove, be sure you get an efficient model that leaves very little ash and releases very little soot. These stoves are not suitable for all homes, so discuss your needs with a heating professional before deciding to switch.

Air-Conditioning

Air conditioners keep you cool and also can remove particulate material that circulates in household air and irritates skin. Any air conditioner you install should bring in fresh outside air, not recirculate dirty air already inside the house. Look for one with a high-efficiency particulate air (HEPA) filter. To keep your air conditioner working, check the filter often to be sure it's not clogged with dust. If it is, change it. Clean the heating and air-conditioning coils at least once a year to cut down on the dust circulated by the system.

Air Cleaners

Air cleaners remove particulate pollution from the air. If your skin is especially sensitive to these invisible irritants, you might want to install one. Look for an air cleaner that removes the highest percentage of particles from the volume of air in your living space. The newspaper weather report often includes pollen levels along with the temperature. Knowing the pollen count for each month in your area will help you determine what kind of filter you'll need. Three good choices are available: window filters; small, freestanding units; and large units that clean the air of the entire house.

Window Filters

Window-size pollen filters get rid of about 96 percent of pollutants carried into your house by breezes. These filters are inexpensive, energy-efficient, and good for individual rooms during the warmer months. In some geographic areas, their use can be restricted to those days when the pollen count is high. The filters also keep out insects, rain, and wind while minimizing noise. They are available at home improvement or hardware stores.

Small, Freestanding Units

Small, freestanding units are fine if the cubic area of air to be cleaned is, for example, a standard-size bedroom. If you get a portable air cleaner, place it so that it's near a specific polluting source and cleaned air is forced into the occupied area. Be sure the air inlet and outlet are not blocked by walls, furniture, or other obstructions. Small units tend to be noisy. Check the sound level of the motor to be sure it won't keep you awake.

Large Units

If you need an air cleaner for the entire house, have a large unit installed at your home's air intake unit. Because they're expensive and affect the air you breathe when you're at home, it's important to take special care in choosing one. Here are some things to discuss with a professional:

- Ion generators and electronic air cleaners may produce ozone, particularly if they are not properly installed and maintained. Ozone can irritate your lungs.

- Be sure that the gases and odors from particles collected are not redispersed into the air.
- The odor of tobacco smoke is due largely to gases in the smoke rather than the particles. Thus, you may smell a tobacco odor even when the smoke particles have been removed.
- Some devices scent the air to mask odors, which may lead you to believe that the odor-causing pollutants have been removed.
- Ion generators, especially those that do not contain a collector, may stain walls and other surfaces.
- Maintenance costs, such as costs for the replacement of filters, may be significant. You should consider these costs in addition to the initial cost of purchase. In general, the most effective units are also the most expensive.

Humidifiers

Indoor humidity of 50 to 55 percent is most comfortable for people with eczema. If you live in a hot, dry, desert area, you probably should invest in a humidifier as well as an air conditioner. If you live in an area with cold winters in a house with forced-air heating, using a humidifier during winter months will help keep your skin from getting too dry. You can get a small, freestanding humidifier for your bedroom to help with this problem. Place it near your bed, so that for a third of the day, at least, you'll be in a well-humidified environment. A central unit will keep the entire house humidified, but it may also create a problem with mold.

Vacuum Cleaning

A good vacuum cleaner can rid your home of much of the dust, mold, mites, pollens, ash, and other invisible particles that can penetrate your skin. Vacuum cleaners differ widely in how much dust they release into the air. If your vacuum cleaner is old, leaks, and is not likely to be fixed by a thorough overhaul, replace it. If you have a good vacuum cleaner and aren't in the house when it's used, it may not be worth getting a special machine. However, if you are doing the vacuuming, either give the job to someone else or get a new machine.

It helps to know what irritates your skin. If pollen is the problem, you don't need as efficient a machine as if you react to dust mite droppings. If you do react to dust mites, look for a vacuum cleaner with guaranteed filtering of objects as small as 0.3 micrometer, with an efficiency rating of 99.97 percent. Here are some more things to keep in mind when shopping for a new vacuum cleaner:

- Avoid water-filled cleaners. They spread aerosols of dust.
- Be careful when selecting a bagless vacuum cleaner. They're difficult to empty without spreading a lot of dust. Even if you empty them outdoors, a cloud of dust is liable to cover your clothes. Mites in the dust will be spread to everything that comes into contact with the clothes you were wearing.
- A central vacuum cleaner is an excellent idea, especially if it's installed while the house is being built. The dust should be piped to a container located outside your living space.

Invisible Irritants: Dust Mites and Mold

Animal dander and mold spores linger in the air. Dust mite and cockroach droppings collect in carpets or bedding, becoming airborne when disturbed. Their concentration increases in confined areas, like houses. Moisture encourages the growth of mold and dust mites. Eczema allows these tiny particles to penetrate the skin's barrier, which can make eczema worse. Mold can be eliminated by wiping down surfaces with a diluted chlorine bleach solution (like Clorox). Let it stand for 5 minutes, then rinse.

Dust mites are microscopic bugs that feed on human and pet dander. Their droppings cause skin irritation in some people. The steps to keep their numbers down will also decrease the amount of other invisible irritants in the air. Dust mites thrive in warm, moist environments, such as the interior of mattresses and pillows or wall-to-wall carpets and drapes. Each week, humans shed about ⅕ ounce of dead skin (dander), which can sustain 100,000 to 10 million mites. If your pillow is several years old, approximately 10 percent of the weight could be mites and their droppings.

Modern technology has created paradise for dust mites. Central heating keeps homes warm all year, and the invention of the vacuum cleaner made wall-to-wall carpeting practical. Add tightly insulated homes, and you have created the perfect environment for dust mites. If you want to see what the population of dust mites is in your home, you can get a home diagnostic kit. Acarex, a dipstick test for mite feces, is available in most pharmacies.

If you do react to mite droppings, you'll want to create a mite-free home—or at least a mite-free room where you can go to recover from flares. If you're going to chose one room as a miteless sanctuary, your bedroom would be the obvious choice.

- To get rid of dust mites that live in your bedding, wrap your pillows and mattress in impermeable covers. The mites will be trapped without food and will subsequently die.

- The covers need to be dustproof, permeable to water vapor, comfortable, and safe for children.
- Pillow covers must completely surround the pillow and be zipped closed.
- The same type of cover is available for mattresses; however, studies have shown that plastic sheets that leave the mattress bottom uncovered work just as well as those that wrap all the way around.

The types of covers available, in order of preference, are as follows:

- Tightly woven cloth, which is soft and "breathes."
- Electrostatic air-filter fiber layer under cloth. This is a two-ply fabric, one side of which is plain cloth, the other of which has a statically charged layer that binds and traps mites and dust.
- Polyurethane cloth, which is woven on one side and shiny plastic on the other. The plastic forms an impermeable barrier.
- Plastic fiber that has been heated and compressed, such as high-density polyethylene. It's inexpensive, but the quality and durability are poor.
- Polyethylene sheets, which are cheap and very effective because they are impermeable to mites. However, they are noisy and they trap moisture, which is especially bad if you live in a humid environment.

Wash all bedcoverings every 2 weeks in water of at least 130 degrees F. If hot water will damage the fabric, freeze it for 24 hours and then wash it at a lower temperature. Wash pillow covers weekly. Wipe plastic pillow covers daily with a damp cloth. Dust mites don't like pillows made of synthetics like Hollofil or Dacron, and they can be washed in very hot water. Wash mattress pads once a month in water of at least 130 degrees F.

Furnishings

Wall Coverings

Paint is preferable to wallpaper because it's more easily cleaned and doesn't attract dust. Wooden paneling is fine as long as it doesn't trap moisture behind it. Choose water-based paints over oil-based paints, as they don't emit as many VOCs and are less irritating to your skin.

Window Dressings

Vertical blinds or shades don't collect as much dust as fabrics and are easy to clean. If you have curtains or drapes, clean them once a month. When buying drapes or curtains, check the fiber content to be sure they're not made from fiberglass.

Carpets

If you react to dust mites, get rid of wall-to-wall carpets. They're havens for mites and also collect pollen, dust, and dander. The most powerful vacuum cleaners are no match for the capacity of wall-to-wall carpets to absorb invisible irritants. While steam cleaning kills mites, it leaves the underside of your carpet warm and wet—the ideal environment for repopulation with mites and mold. Instead of wall-to-wall carpets, buy throw rugs that can be washed in water hot enough to kill mites. When you buy rugs, check the fiber content. Wool and fiberglass both release tiny fibers that can irritate your skin.

Upholstered Furniture

Dust mites love soft, fuzzy fabrics. It's best to have furniture made of wood, or covered in plastic, vinyl, or leather. However, if you do have cloth upholstery, vacuum it weekly. Wash throw pillows, afghans, and other fabric objects in hot water (130 degrees F) twice a month.

You can also treat fabrics with an antimite solution. Acarosan and Allergy Control Solution are two products that contain benzoyl benzoate and tannic acid, neither of which is harmful to humans. Benzoyl benzoate, the "miticide," kills 99 percent of mites. Tannic acid doesn't kill mites, but it alters their proteins so their droppings are no longer irritating.

Other tips for controlling dust mites:

- Keep the door to your bedroom (if that's your sanctuary) closed.
- Keep clutter to a minimum. Dust bunnies and dander are picked up by air currents and dropped behind knickknacks. These tiny piles of dander provide a feast for dust mites. After dinner, they add their sticky feces to the pile. When the pile dries, the slightest breeze picks it up and scatters it throughout your room.
- Wash stuffed animals, throw pillows, and any other stuffed objects in hot water every 2 weeks.
- Clean curtains once a month, following the manufacturer's instructions. Don't let pets into your bedroom. Letting your pets in just once a week will undo all your best efforts at keeping your bedroom mite-free.

• • • •

While dust mites are found in every home, other bugs show up only in certain areas. The northeastern United States is a favored habitat for bedbugs. Fleas prefer temperate climates. The bites of both creatures can cause serious reactions in some people with eczema. When I see patients whose eczema gets better when they go on trips, I always ask them to check for these bugs at home. Their presence doesn't mean poor housekeeping. Bedbugs are easily transported via furniture, suitcases, or other objects brought into your home. Since they are very clever at staying out of sight, you probably won't notice them, but you will be able to see the bites on your body in the morning. If so, check your bed at night to see if the bedbugs have come out for a meal. Fleas are more noticeable since they're active during the day and tend to hop about. Pets are the most common vehicle for fleas to get into your house.

If you are following the steps to keep your home free from dust mites, this will help in keeping your home free of other pests as well. Both fleas and bedbugs are visible to the human eye, so if you see them or suspect their presence, call a professional exterminator to get rid of them.

Houseplants—Nature's Helpers

Scientists at NASA performed several studies to see whether plants absorb pollutants from their environments. They found that houseplants did indeed remove unwanted and unhealthy household chemicals such as formaldehyde (released by particleboard, carpets, cleaning products, and cooking fuels) and benzene (found in paints, plastics, and detergents).

"Plants take substances out of the air through the tiny openings in their leaves," according to Dr. Bill Wolverton, formerly a senior research scientist at NASA's John C. Stennis Space Center in Mississippi. "But research in our laboratories has determined that plant leaves, roots, and soil bacteria are all important in removing trace levels of toxic vapors." While plants can't do it all, they can help. In addition, they're soothing to live with, beautiful to look at, and relaxing to tend. Here are the top ten plants for removing formaldehyde, benzene, and carbon monoxide from your air:

- Bamboo palm *(Chamaedorea seifrizii)*
- Chinese evergreen *(Aglaonema modestum)*
- English ivy *(Hedera helix)*
- Gerbera daisy *(Gerbera jamesonii)*
- Janet Craig *(Dracaena "Janet Craig")*
- Marginata *(Dracaena marginata)*
- Mass cane/corn plant *(Dracaena massangeana)*
- Mother-in-law's tongue *(Sansevieria laurentii)*
- Pot mum *(Chrysanthemum morifolium)*
- Peace lily *(Spathiphyllum "mauna loa")*
- Warneckii (*Dracaena "warneckii")*

A large part of staying eczema-free is controlling environmental factors that irritate your skin. There have been many instances where just changing things around the house has been enough to cut down on flares and keep skin soft and clear.

Chapter Nine

MANAGING ADULT LIFE

Eczema is an unwanted, constant companion. It is with you at work, on dates, and at home. Learning to live with eczema requires more than careful medical treatments. This chapter tells you how to cope when eczema shows up when you least want to deal with it.

ECZEMA AT WORK

Skin rash is the second most common workplace illness (after back pain), which means about one-third of all work-related health problems is due to rashes. Hand eczema alone costs the United States billions of dollars for absenteeism, lost income, retraining, rehabilitation, medical bills, legal bills, and disability. This reflects only reported cases. It doesn't include many with hand eczema who don't report it, nor does it include those who suffer flares from job-related stress. Work doesn't cause eczema, but it can make it worse.

Not all occupational rashes are eczema. Some are the result of industrial chemicals that damage even the healthiest skin. However, if you have eczema, you are at greater risk for reactions than those without it. Eighty percent of work-related problems involve the hands because they are used for virtually every kind of job.

Occupations where the hands are constantly immersed in water or chemicals have the highest incidence of problems with hand eczema, while white-collar office jobs have the lowest incidence. The occupation with the greatest number of those with hand eczema is housekeeping, especially if it's combined with infant care. Other occupations, like veterinary medicine, have an equally high incidence, but there are fewer veterinarians than housewives.

Having eczema doesn't necessarily mean that you have to avoid certain careers, but it does mean you'll need to be well educated about the disorder and how your work affects it. A recent study in Finland looked at 1,008 adults who had developed work-related hand eczema. Those with the greatest understanding of eczema were able to manage their skin and their jobs just fine. I believe education is the key. If you know what impact eczema has on your career, you can take steps to prevent problems.

At the same time, it helps to be realistic. Discuss your career options with your doctor. If you have severe eczema, you are more likely to have trouble in those careers that require constant exposure to chemicals. If you want to be a nurse, for example, but you and your doctor agree that frequent hand washing is out of the question, consider aspects of nursing that don't require intense wear and tear on your skin, such as research, public health policy, or administration.

The following occupations are those that present the greatest risk of hand eczema.

Hairdressing

Hairdressers' hands are exposed to irritation from a variety of sources: hair burrowing into the skin, frequent hand immersion in hot, soapy water, and the use of chemicals to style and color hair.

Food Industry

If you work in a busy restaurant, you'll spend hours every day doing things that bother eczema, such as cutting vegetables, working with juices and sauces, cleaning kitchen implements and dishware, and kneading bread. You're also likely to be washing your hands frequently, using very hot, soapy water.

Automobile Repair

Each day you'll be up to your elbows in oils, brake fluid, transmission fluid, and coolant. Then you'll scrub them off with solvents, abrasive brushes and soaps, and lots of very hot water. This is terrible treatment for hand eczema.

Health Care

If you are a doctor, nurse, physical therapist, medical assistant, dentist, dental hygienist, veterinarian, veterinary assistant, or other health care worker, there can be many problems for eczema:

- Constant hand washing
- Irritation from gloves
- Exposure to infectious blood and body fluids
- Exposure to infections
- Vaccination requirements

Animal Handlers

In addition to veterinarians, this includes animal control officers, animal trainers, zoo workers, game wardens, wildlife zoologists, biologists who work with animals, farmers, and ranchers. Animal dander, feathers, and saliva may irritate your skin. Further irritation is caused by frequent hand washing and improper use of gloves.

Brick- and Plasterwork

Cement is alkaline and can cause severe burns or irritation to the skin. Anyone who works with cement on a daily basis is at risk.

Arts and Crafts

Fine arts professionals, musical instrument craftspeople, surfboard makers, sports equipment manufacturers, and cabinetmakers all work with chemicals that can exacerbate hand eczema.

• • •

In fact, there are very few jobs that never involve exposure to something that can bother eczema. So here are some steps you can take to protect yourself:

- Make sure your health and disability insurance covers all aspects of eczema.
- Make sure your employer follows OSHA (Occupational Safety and Health Administration) guidelines for all its employees.
- Talk to your future colleagues about the level of care the organization has for its employees.
- Find out if your employer takes protective measures for its employees in the workplace.

- Find out if protective personal clothing is available.
- Find out if the environment is clean and free of contamination.
- Make sure suitable skin care products are made available to you to protect your skin.
- Make sure there is an MSDS (materials safety data sheet) on all hazardous materials so you or your doctor can determine your level of risk should you suffer an exposure.
- Make sure there are emergency showers in case you're accidentally splashed.
- Find out if there are alternative compounds that your company can use that are less hazardous.
- Ask if your employer is receptive to safety suggestions.
- Ask if you'll be trained to do another task if you can't continue your original job because of eczema.

Gloves: Your Best Protection

Because eczema at work tends to involve the hands, gloves are your best protection. Gloves may help you keep a career you wouldn't be able to pursue otherwise. Like other aspects of eczema, education is crucial. Know what each type of glove can protect you from, and be sure you have the right glove for the job at hand. For example, in the hospital I use latex gloves. I know that petrolatum can weaken the latex so that it's no longer impermeable. I also know that iodine discolors latex but doesn't damage it. Your employer should be able to tell you what exposure a particular glove can withstand and for how long. You can also get this information from the glove manufacturer. Here are some problems to be aware of when wearing gloves:

- Watch out for punctures from needles or other sharp objects.

- If the glove is permeable and your hand is exposed to a hazardous substance, this is doubly dangerous. First, the substance penetrates through the glove to your skin. Then the glove keeps the substance from escaping anywhere but into your skin.
- Gloves trap moisture and heat, which may make your hands itch. It's also a perfect environment for bacteria, so in addition to encouraging eczema, your skin might get infected. To avoid the buildup of moisture, use a glove with an absorbent liner, or wear thin cotton gloves under the work gloves. Take frequent breaks to air your hands. If you still have problems, I recommend Zeasorb AF powder. It absorbs excess moisture and has antibacterial and antifungal properties. You can buy it without a prescription.
- Gloves interfere with your sense of touch and hand mobility. This is especially true when you wear two pairs of gloves. The upside is that you'll eventually adapt to the diminished sensitivity and mobility, and after a while, you won't even notice a difference between your gloved hand and your ungloved hand.
- For the best protection, gloves are superior to barrier creams. The creams are only partially protective, and only for a limited time. If you use Gloves in a Bottle®, keep in mind that your hands are not fully protected from irritants.

Skin Care Products for Work

Skin care products are second only to gloves in protecting your hands. At home and at work, use only the best. If your employer is using inferior products or those inappropriate for your skin, make a special request for the items you need. You'll need both cleaning products and hand creams. If your employer doesn't want to bother with special orders, see if you'd be reimbursed if you buy your own. If you have to pay for your own products, check with your tax adviser to determine if the cost is deductible. Get travel sizes to put in your handbag, briefcase, glove compartment, desk drawer, or pocket.

Be sure that the hand creams you use are appropriate to the type of exposure you are experiencing. There are specialized skin preparations that counterbalance different kinds of irritants.

- For **water-soluble compounds** such as cleansing agents, disinfectants, and coolants, you need a thick barrier cream with a high lipid content after each exposure. *Impruv* is one brand that works.
- For **alkaline chemicals** such as ammonia-based cleaners or cement, use a thick barrier cream with a high lipid content that has a neutral or slightly acidic pH. Gloves in a Bottle is an example of this type of cream.
- For **organic solvents and oils** used by painters or mechanics, you need a water-soluble, film-forming polymer to protect your skin. Try Proteque or Theraseal.
- If your skin is constantly dirty or if you're working with agents that stick to your skin like **oil, adhesives, resins, and paints,** apply an emulsifying cream to your skin before working. To clean up, avoid harsh cleansers. Try dissolving the substance with mineral or cooking oil first.
- If you work with **rough or abrasive substances** such as sand, steel wool, or glass, you're likely to get microcracks in your skin, which will allow irritants through. Consider using Colloidin before working with these materials.
- If your exposure is to **sun,** be sure to wear sunscreen. Mechanical sunscreens work best. These contain iron oxide, zinc oxide, or titanium oxide as their principal pro-

tective agent. Don't forget that clothing and sunglasses are also mechanical sun barriers.

Hand Washing Techniques

When washing your hands, be aware that even water can deplete natural moisturizers. Soaps and detergents dissolve natural oils in water as they remove dirt and grime. This damages the barrier and leaves the skin vulnerable to irritants, which can worsen eczema. Use the following guidelines to keep hands clean with minimal damage to the skin's barrier:

- Use a cleanser appropriate to what you're trying to wash away.
- Use the mildest cleanser that does the job. Here are some acceptable ingredients to look for: Very gentle—alkyl polyglycosides, ethoxylated fatty acid glycerides, betaine derivatives, sulfosuccinates, ethoxylated fatty alcohols, or isethionates. Less gentle—fatty alcohol ether sulfates or alkylolamides.
- Wash only when necessary. There are times that just patting the hands or gently rinsing the hands with water is enough.
- For those who need frequent washings in hot water, like medical staff, try rinseless cleansers that contain isopropyl alcohol. It's often less irritating to eczema skin.
- Use a moist towelette to gently wipe away grime and debris.
- Avoid cleansers with harsh detergents or irritants. The following are some ingredients to avoid—alpha-olefin sulfonates, secondary alkane sufonates, alkylbenzene sulfonates, or fatty alcohol sulfates.
- Use hand cream after every cleansing.

Coworkers

When dealing with coworkers, understand that most people probably want to help but may not know how. The policy of speaking openly applies not only to your family but also to those you work with.

Eczema flares may interfere with some work tasks. You may need to rearrange your schedule for doctor visits, special treatments, or even hospitalization. Discuss your needs with your employer. Don't forget that it is illegal for you to be fired because of ill health. If you feel you are being harassed on the job because of your illness, contact your union representative or your state legislator about your rights. Employers must make "reasonable accommodations" on your behalf to allow you to do your work. If you suffer from eczema to the extent that any of your major life activities is impaired, you may qualify for protection under the Americans with Disabilities Act. If speaking to your employer is not effective, you may require the services of an attorney.

INSURANCE COVERAGE

Dealing with Insurance Companies

It's demoralizing and infuriating to pay regular premiums to a health insurance company only to learn when you need treatment that the company doesn't, or refuses to, cover it. Skin disorders are often considered cosmetic, not medical, problems, and some insurance companies routinely deny the claims. Sometimes you have to submit the bill several times before receiving reimbursement. Here are some ways to redress this outrage:

- Call your insurance carrier and ask if eczema treatment is covered in the policy.

- If treatment is covered by your insurer, ask what portion of the payment you'll be responsible for (the copayment) as well as the maximum the company will allow for ongoing treatment. Also, ask if the coverage provides for outpatient and inpatient treatment.
- Every time you speak with an insurance company representative, write down his or her name, the time of your call, the date, and the information you receive. If you get a verbal agreement for coverage, request that the representative send it to you in writing. If you don't receive it, follow up with additional requests until you get it.
- Check with your doctor about his or her experience with insurance coverage for eczema treatments and how other patients have dealt with their claims. He or she may be aware of strategies that have worked for others or of insurance plans that will cover these services.
- In petitioning for coverage of a specific eczema treatment, provide your insurance company with well-documented information supporting its effectiveness. Include articles from medical journals, corroborating data from your doctor, and a description of your own experiences with the condition.
- If your insurance company denies you reimbursement for a treatment, have your doctor write a letter of medical necessity explaining the importance of the treatment. This should be accompanied by a letter of your own, explaining what happens when you don't get therapy and, possibly, how it might end up costing the insurance company even more to treat complications from delayed therapy.
- If treatment payment is denied after you have tried all these strategies, keep fighting. Inform your insurance company that you are prepared to fight for coverage of eczema treatment and that you will contact your em-

ployer's human resources representative, your elected state representatives, your state's insurance committee, and an attorney, if necessary. Then do so.

- If you should leave your job for any reason, be sure you continue your insurance under the Consolidated Omnibus Budget Reconciliation Act (COBRA). This provision gives you the right to participate in your former employer's group insurance on your own for up to eighteen months after you leave your job. It may be expensive, but if you're unable to work or you have difficulty finding another job, it's definitely worth it.

It's unlikely that your insurance will deny coverage of a second or third opinion. But they may deny coverage for off-label use of drugs (the practice of prescribing a drug approved by the Food and Drug Administration [FDA] for one condition to treat a different condition), for experimental treatments, or for preexisting conditions (which may be a problem if you have to change insurance carriers).

In some cases, you may need the services of an attorney who specializes in patient advocacy or insurance problems. Call your local bar association or a nearby law school, or look under "Lawyer Referral Service" in the Yellow Pages of your local telephone directory. You and your lawyer may try a couple of simple strategies to solve these problems. You can write to your insurance company, explaining that you intend to contact a lawyer. You can have your lawyer send the company a letter stating that he or she intends to press a claim on your behalf. Sometimes that's all that's needed.

Be persistent in pressing your claim. An insurance company may try to wait you out, stalling until you give up and stop fighting. If they know you are serious and unlikely to give up, they're more likely to accommodate your request. Talk to your human resources representative at work about any insurance problems. These are the people who contract with insurance companies for the benefit of employees. If your needs as an employee are not being met, the human resources representative can bring that up directly with the insurance company. Your company may even consider switching to a new insurance carrier when it's time to renew enrollment.

In addition to pursuing the insurance company directly, don't hesitate to call your local media and go public with your insurance problem. Dramatic policy reversals in the last decade have occurred when patients have brought their plights to public attention.

Spread the Word

Some of the most significant social changes in history have come about because ordinary people have gotten angry enough to fight back. Spurred to action by the inequities of a system that seems more concerned with the bottom line than the needs of the individual, they have gone public with their grievances by lobbying legislators for everything from wheelchair ramps to nonsmoking workplaces. In doing so, they've enhanced their own and other people's lives immeasurably.

To effect change in your community, start with a local eczema support group. If there isn't one, ask your dermatologist to help you start one and ask him or her to participate by speaking to interested groups. The more people involved, the stronger your message. However, even if you find yourself on the front lines alone, don't stop. One voice can do a lot.

Alone or with a group, prepare your attack. The Internet probably has most of what you'll need. Collect statistics on the cost of eczema, the number of people with eczema, research dollars spent compared with other disorders, the quality of eczema research, and anything else you can think of. If possible, put it all together in a nice package that you can distribute to insurance companies, state and federal legislators, medical schools, and the press.

Then start calling. Contact medical schools to see how much training medical students get on the cause and treatment of eczema. My medical school spent less than one hour discussing eczema. If little information is given to students, offer to send your packet. Ask if they'd like the dermatologists in your group to give special presentations on eczema.

Contact the local offices of your state and federal legislators. Keep in mind that these are the people who set the laws for Medicare and state medical insurance programs. They have tremendous influence on how and what is covered. Once the government covers an illness or treatment, private insurers follow suit. Your representatives also want to stay in office, so they're willing to listen, and if they see a program that will result in votes, they'll be grateful to you for bringing it to their attention.

Legislators also vote on allocating funds for research and writing laws to punish or control the insurance industry. Send e-mails to all legislators in every state urging them to increase the amount of money the government allocates for research into the causes of, and effective treatment for, eczema. If the government can allocate money to study why people fall in love or why inmates want to escape from prison, it can certainly find the funds to investigate this lifelong condition. You can even call the White House Opinion Line and tell the operator you are concerned about the lack of research in eczema.

Become media savvy. Make an appointment to see the editor of your local newspaper or the producer of a local television or radio show to suggest a news story or feature about eczema. Explain the importance and widespread nature of the condition and describe your own experience. Bring along the packet of information you've put together.

Speak with others who have eczema about what you have learned, where you found treatment, and how you dealt with your insurance company, among other issues. This will empower them and possibly inspire them to speak with others. Join the National Eczema Association for Science and Education (NEASE) or your local eczema support group. Start a fundraising project for eczema research and let the local media know about your efforts. Write to special interest health organizations and encourage them to publish information about eczema. The more publicity this condition receives, the better.

TRAVELING WITH ECZEMA

There's no reason not to go anywhere you want, as long as you go prepared. Learn about the area you are visiting. Determine the local health and vaccination requirements. Find out if there are any health advisories for your destination. Often this information can be gleaned from the U.S. State Department, or from your physician's office.

Find out about the climate and take appropriate attire with you. Also, knowing about the weather will help you determine what to expect from your eczema. For example, if cold, dry weather worsens your eczema and you're going to the Rocky Mountains to ski, you can expect an eczema flare. Alternatively, if you tend to get fungal infections and these worsen your eczema, be prepared when traveling to the tropics.

If you are going somewhere that is likely to worsen your eczema, be sure to pack the appropriate types and quantities of medication and nonmedical treatments that you need. This is particularly important if you're traveling to remote areas. Keep medications or prescriptions in your carry-on luggage when traveling. Once at your destination, carry them with you at all times. Be sure your prescription medication is in clearly labeled containers. You don't want authorities along your journey to confiscate your medications because you don't have proof that the medication was prescribed by your doctor.

Take extra precautions with cuts, scrapes, and wounds. It's one thing to be at home and have a skin infection—it's quite another to be at a campsite or in a remote village where you don't speak the language. Be aggressive about treating problems early. At the slightest sign of a flare or infection, begin therapy. Don't let a minor irritation develop into something that puts you in the hospital.

Buy travel insurance. This is relatively inexpensive and can be purchased through your travel agent or on the Internet. The cost of the insurance is based upon the cost of the trip. You can often get coverage for travel costs as well as medical costs in case of emergency. The medical costs can be particularly helpful in foreign countries, where access to quality facilities may be scarce or restricted to local residents. With good travel insurance, you can get transportation to a medical facility, care at a clinic or hospital covered, and emergency evacuation back home if necessary.

Take your own cleansers with you. Hotel soaps, moisturizers, conditioners, and lotions may not be appropriate for you. You can purchase travel-size bottles (Nalgene brand bottles come in all sizes and are leakproof) to carry your own skin care products in quantities that are just right for your trip. If you're taking an extended trip, you can't take an infinite stock of materials with you. Jot down the names of skin care products that you use, and ask shopkeepers and pharmacists where you can purchase supplies locally.

When you choose a place to stay, look for the following:

- Nonsmoking rooms
- No-pet rooms
- Nonirritating bedding (natural fabrics, no synthetics, no wool)
- Adjustable temperature in the room
- Quiet (rest is very important for eczema)

If you're going to indulge yourself at a spa, do some investigating before you sign up. Make sure the staff are accredited or licensed and that they practice good hygiene. Find out if any treatments are damaging to your sensitive skin, such as manicures, pedicures, treatments with abrasive materials, or hot stones. If these are offered, be sure to avoid them.

Seaweed wraps and mud baths don't seem to bother eczema. Tar treatments and saltwater treatments actually appear to help it.

In deciding where to go on your vacation, consider a trip to the ocean. Sun and salt water can do wonders for your eczema, but check with your doctor before you make your reservations. Take at least 1 week and soak in the ocean for at least 20 minutes a day. When you get out, cover up. Don't try to get a tan. One week, particularly in the middle of winter if you live in a northern climate, is as good as weeks and weeks of home care and medication. If you like inland salt seas, try the Salt Lake in Utah or the Salton Sea in California. In the Middle East, the Dead Sea is a favorite.

SEXUAL HEALTH

Menstruation

Some women report that eczema worsens the week preceding their periods, while at the same time rendering treatments less effective. With the onset of the menstrual flow, the flares die down and treatments are once again effective. If you experience a similar problem, it will help to plan ahead. Keep a flare calendar so you can anticipate them. If you treat your eczema aggressively before the flare hits, its impact will be blunted and the duration shortened.

Conception

The FDA gives a letter code to prescription medications to indicate their safety during conception and pregnancy. The drugs listed here are only for eczema. Check with your doctor for other medications that may be harmful. To be absolutely safe, both parents should generally avoid the use of internal (taken by mouth or injected) prescription medications for eczema when trying to conceive a child. The following eczema treatments require precautions.

Medication	Pregnancy Category
Topical Steroids	C: Avoid unless necessary. No clear evidence of birth defects.
Cyclosporine	C: Avoid unless necessary. No clear evidence of birth defects.
Methotrexate	X: Absolutely avoid. Even small doses can cause birth defects in the first trimester.
UVB	B: Safe for the fetus during pregnancy. However, may cause dark brown spots to develop on the face in pregnant women (melasma).
Emollients	A: Safe during pregnancy.

Methotrexate (MTX) is a potent drug used to treat severe or disabling eczema. It's capable of causing miscarriages or fetal malformations. Men and women should discontinue using MTX at least twelve weeks before trying to conceive. It poses little or no risk to pregnancies that occur after it has been discontinued. MTX does not harm a man's or a woman's long-term potential of conceiving a normal child. However, it may lower a man's sperm count temporarily. According to a few reports, men who have taken MTX during the time of conception have fathered healthy children.

Cyclosporine (brand name Neoral) is another potent drug used for cases of severe or disabling eczema. Based on a relatively small number of cases, cyclosporine does not appear to pose a major fetal risk for pregnant women. A worldwide registry of transplant patients (cyclosporine suppresses the immune system and so is used primarily in organ transplant cases) treated with the drug during pregnancy did not show an increased rate of birth defects, although low birth weight and premature birth were traced to cyclosporine use. Cyclosporine should be used during pregnancy only if the potential benefit to the mother outweighs the potential risk to the fetus. The drug is not known to affect a man's fertility.

Pregnancy

How pregnancy affects a woman with eczema has not been adequately studied; therefore, there are no reliable research results. However, there have been studies on how medications or treatments affect the fetus. For pregnant women with mild eczema, over-the-counter remedies such as emollients are considered to be safe. Check with your doctor if you have any doubts or questions.

Topical steroids are classified as category C. Package inserts advise that these treatments should be used only if their benefits to the mother outweigh potential risks to their fetus. Therefore, if topical steroids are required, the amount applied to the skin should be limited. Superpotent steroids should be used only if essential, and occlusion, or use of wraps, should be minimized. Studies of pregnant women treated with oral steroids have not found an increase in birth defects, despite animal studies suggesting they cause an increased incidence of cleft palate. Work closely with your doctor when taking any medications during pregnancy.

When eczema is sufficiently severe and topical treatments aren't helping, light therapy may be considered. Treatment with UVB may be as safe as sunlight, but sunscreen should be used on the face to prevent skin damage.

Breast-Feeding

Eczema on nipples will not harm a nursing infant; however, it may cause the mother discomfort. Since breast-feeding is so important for the health a newborn, try to treat the discomfort rather than discontinue breast-feeding. Moisturize the nipples with thick emollients or moisturizers. If this isn't enough, ask your doctor for suggestions. UVB is generally acceptable as an eczema therapy for women who are breast-feeding.

Topical medications should not be used on the nipples. Also, there is a slight chance some drugs will be absorbed by the body through the skin and get into the mother's milk. This is especially true if large areas of the skin are covered with medication. Work closely with your doctor to determine what is acceptable topical therapy while nursing. All systemic medications for eczema should be avoided when breast-feeding. These agents could be secreted in the breast milk and ingested by the infant.

Genital Area

Eczema of the genital area can be difficult to diagnose and treat. If you are experiencing redness and irritation, remember that in addition to eczema, you may have other conditions. As long as eczema is the only problem, intercourse, so long as it does not cause irritation, is not prohibited. Sometimes lubricants are recommended, particularly if the skin is quite dry and irritated.

Eczema on the pubis is treated similarly to eczema on the scalp. While you are showering, the area may be treated with a medicated shampoo that contains tar or *salicylic acid,* both safe for the pubic area. A steroid cream may be applied afterward. Care must be taken to limit exposure of the genitals to UV light because this skin burns more easily and the risk of skin cancer is increased. Home UV light therapy is not advised owing to the risk of burning this sensitive skin.

Eczema of the upper thighs often consists of one large patch or many small patches that are red and scaly. The usual treatments include topical applications of emollients or steroids, or ultraviolet light therapy. Mild or low-strength topical steroids are generally used to treat the thigh—superpotent topical steroids can produce stretch marks if overused.

Eczema is less scaly and more red in the creases between the thigh and groin. The skin may have fissures (cracks). It may be necessary to have a skin sample examined under a microscope to determine if a yeast or fungal infection is also present.

Eczema of the vulva often appears as a smooth, nonscaly redness that usually is quite itchy. If this sensitive area is irritated by scratching, it may become infected. Scratching also can produce dryness, thickening (lichenification), and further itching of the skin. A doctor needs to determine the cause of the discomfort before treating this area for eczema.

Genital eczema affects both circumcised and uncircumcised males. Eczema of the penis may appear as many small red patches on the tip or shaft. The skin may be red and scaly, or it may be red and smooth. Low-strength topical steroids such as hydrocortisone may be used for very short periods for both female and male patients.

Because genital skin is sensitive and thin, potent steroids should be avoided or used for only a few days at the beginning of treatment. Topical immunomodulators (TIMs) are anti-inflammatory medications that do not cause atrophy of thin genital skin. Tacrolimus (brand name Protopic) or pimecrolimus (brand name Elidel) are two examples of prescription TIMs. They sometimes cause burning and irritation during initial flares, so treatment can be preceded by a few days of mild-potency topical steroids. Skin can become abnormally thin if steroid preparations are used over a long period.

Male patients undergoing any kind of ultraviolet light therapy should protect the penis and the scrotum. Men should wear briefs or athletic supporters to protect their genitals while sunbathing or receiving UV light treatment on other parts of the body. Studies indicate that skin on the male genitals should not be exposed to UV radiation, particularly PUVA (the light-sensitizing drug Psoralen plus UVA light), because of the possibility of an increased risk of skin cancer.

Eczema in the vicinity of the anus is red, may or may not be scaly, and is prone to intense itchiness. It usually responds to emollients and low-strength steroids. Eczema in this area may be confused with yeast or fungal infections, hemorrhoidal itching, psoriasis, scabies, and even pinworm infestations. The presence of these conditions can complicate the treatment of eczema and make the eczema worse. Rectal examinations, skin cultures, and examinations for pinworm can confirm these conditions so they can be treated appropriately.

Genital Itching

Aloe vera gel is a mild, relatively inexpensive product that is effective in relieving itching for some people. Aveeno oilated oatmeal mixed in bathwater is useful for soaking the affected areas, 2 to 3 times a day for 20-minute periods. Oral antihistamines are occasionally prescribed for itching of this area. Over-the-counter lotions with benzocaine should be avoided. Anti-itch preparations containing pramoxine, menthol, or camphor are effective and less likely to cause allergic reactions.

The type of underclothing you wear can also affect itching. Cotton undergarments are preferable to nylon, and tight underwear may aggravate eczema. Formaldehyde, a chemical used in permanent press fabrics, has been shown to be irritating to the skin. Washing new clothes before wearing them may help. Products containing or coated with latex, including some feminine hygiene products, have been reported to irritate eczema in the genital area.

Chapter Ten

MANAGING YOUR EMOTIONS

When I first see adult patients, many of them have struggled so long with eczema that they have lost much of the courage they need to face life. If the eczema involves visible areas like the face and scalp, they don't have the emotional strength to meet new people. This leads to social isolation and loneliness. When the National Eczema Society did a survey in 1996 of eczema sufferers, it found that 86 percent felt self-conscious about their looks. A similar percentage said eczema had negatively affected one or more aspects of their lives, such as job prospects, interviews, promotions, making friends, or finding a mate. Those who had eczema as children remembered the unhappiness of being rejected and teased.

Unlike cancer or heart disease, eczema cannot be hidden. Eczema is rarely life-threatening, so most people, including many doctors, regard it more as a cosmetic problem than a medical condition. In addition to the effect on appearance, the unpredictability of eczema exacts a terrific emotional toll. Flares come without warning and with no way of knowing how long they'll last. The itching interferes with sleep and the ability to think about anything else. Intense itching forces a frenzy of uncontrolled scratching regardless of where you are or what you're doing. Flares can suddenly erupt at work, at a party, or while making love.

Adults with eczema often suffer alone, without emotional support from friends, family, and, most shamefully, the medical profession. A major shortcoming of Western medicine is its failure to address the total impact of disease. The current biomedical model regards the body as if it were a car engine. If something doesn't work, fix it or replace it. Few doctors take the time to understand how disease effects the emotional well-being of their patients. Even fewer take the time to offer help with their patients' distress.

This emotional distress is neither self-indulgent nor an indication of weakness of spirit or mental illness. It's as much a part of the eczema syndrome as itching and rash. Most people agree that professional medical care is important when someone has an itchy, infected rash. At the same time, many of these same people don't think it's important to get professional help for the emotional distress caused by the disorder.

Adding to the misery of eczema sufferers is the persistent myth that eczema is a psychological disorder. In fact, eczema is also called *neurodermatitis* (which means a rash caused by emotions), a misnomer that helps perpetuate the fallacy. Underlying this myth, however, is the reality that emotional distress can trigger a flare. Depression suppresses the immune system, allowing the skin's invaders to prevail over the body's immune response. In eczema, mind and body work together to either conquer the symptoms or make them worse.

In this chapter, I'll discuss the many different emotional issues that my eczema patients face. While there's no magic solution to erase the emotional pain many feel, there are ways to mitigate it. Managing the psychological stress of eczema is as important as a good home care routine for your skin. Combining the two will keep you eczema-free.

CONQUER NEGATIVE FEELINGS

Feelings of helplessness hinder the ability of the immune system to function normally. Believing that you have control over your eczema keeps the immune system functioning as it should. If you have lost your will to fight back, explore assertiveness training. Start with a trip to your library or bookstore to read about the subject. This may be all the information you need. However, if you want to pursue it further, every metropolitan area has assertiveness training classes.

Meanwhile, don't just think about what you'd like to do—do it. Take flying lessons instead of dreaming about the freedom of the blue. Call a person you've been meaning to talk to. As you act more and wish less, you'll be taking charge of your life. Each success will encourage you to try something more. If you hit a stumbling block, figure out how to get around it. Assertiveness training will set you on the path to conquer some common negative feelings people with eczema have. Acknowledging that these feelings exist is step one on the road to overcoming them.

Self-Loathing

Eczema makes some people hate the way they look to the point where they don't want to look at or touch their own skin. One patient bought a sponge on a long handle so she wouldn't have to touch herself when she showered. They hate themselves for having the disorder, and they assume everyone else does, too. Learning to love and respect your own body will encourage good home care, which in turn will lead to less eczema.

Anger

Anger at having eczema can be a normal and healthy reaction if it mobilizes your determination to fight back. Anger becomes dangerous when it's denied and the rage simmers beneath the surface, ready to boil over for the least reason. Acknowledging your anger toward those without eczema for their insensitive remarks, or even toward your parents for passing on your genetic makeup, will make you feel better, even if you do nothing else.

Anger turned inward doesn't fool anyone except yourself. Others see it and back away, leaving you isolated and friendless. You end up killing off the simple pleasures in your life, becoming hardened and embittered. It feels good to express anger, especially if it's been bottled up for a long time. The key is to find ways and settings where you can do it safely and constructively, such as support groups or therapy.

Self-Blame

Blaming yourself for eczema originates with the attitude that the sick person is responsible for having the sickness. If the person were stronger, better, more positive, then he or she wouldn't have the disorder. While you can do a lot to take charge of your eczema, you can't cure it yourself. What you can do is minimize the extent of your flares by arming yourself with information.

Thinking you alone are at fault encourages the idea that you must have brought the disease on yourself—a feeling many eczema patients and parents erroneously hold.

It's a waste of time and energy to ruminate about what caused your eczema. What matters is what you do about your condition now. This includes using every strategy and resource available and exploring every credible treatment possible to manage your condition.

Fear

No one with eczema escapes fear when confronted with the prospect of having a lifelong illness. Fear is an appropriate reaction to uncertainty. You don't know when a flare will start or how long it will last. You don't know if you'll have an eczema-free vacation or a ruined one. Neither you nor the medical profession knows everything there is to learn about eczema.

Keeping in mind that uncertainty promotes fear, self-education is the best way to fight it. Read everything you can find about eczema. Sort facts from fiction, then cling to the truth. Listen to your dermatologist and work with him or her to find the best course of treatment for you. You may not always be eczema-free, but you won't be afraid to face it.

Stress

Stress is not just an unpleasant feeling; it has a profound effect on the severity of flares and on the health of your entire body. As mentioned earlier, negative emotions suppress the body's immune system. Since eczema is a disorder of the skin's immune function, eczema sufferers already have immune problems that are multiplied by added stress.

Stress hormones make the skin's blood vessels sticky in order to attract white blood cells to an area your body thinks is under attack. The white cells are pushed through the vessel walls and go to work finding invaders, calling in reserves, and, by their activity, triggering inflammation. This is the same process created by invaders penetrating the skin from the outside. When someone with eczema is stressed, inflammation can attack both from inside your body and from your environment.

A major source of stress among eczema sufferers is repressed feelings. Those who don't allow themselves to feel the pain of eczema will be more likely to develop physical symptoms. If you need to cry, go ahead and do so. Give yourself permission to feel even the most upsetting of emotions. Getting it out and being honest with yourself will be therapeutic. Feeling bad won't make you sick, but pretending to feel good when you don't could.

The greater the role that stress plays in your eczema, the greater the benefit you'll get from stress management and psychological intervention techniques. Even small reductions in stress can lead to tremendous improvements in overall well-being and the reduction of symptoms.

As difficult as it may seem sometimes, stay positive. Make a list of the good things in your life and put it where you can see it often. List

- things about yourself that you enjoy.
- accomplishments you are proud of.
- aspects of your life that make you happy.
- people who bring joy to your life.
- activities you like doing.

Take extra care of yourself when your eczema is out of control. Pamper yourself by putting your needs first. Let those who are close to you know what you need. Include them in your life, let them help, and let them know how important they are to you.

Depression

When negative emotions take over, the end result is clinical depression. This is not just feeling sad. Clinical depression changes your body's chemistry and must be treated by a physician. In eczema, when itching gets worse, depression deepens. Depression lowers the itch threshold and so starts a downward spiral. Diagnosing depression is important for overall health and for alleviating eczema symptoms. It's easy to misinterpret depression and blame feeling down on the weather, a broken appliance, or an upsetting conversation. There is a difference between reactive depression—sadness that results from a particular event in your life, which is short-lived—and clinical depression, which doesn't go away on its own.

To assess depression, ask yourself the following. Have you had

- chronic feelings of sadness or despair?
- loss of appetite?
- overeating?
- oversleeping?
- insomnia?
- withdrawal from friends, family, coworkers?
- atypical irritability or anger?
- inability to concentrate?
- little or no interest in sex?
- lack of normal energy?
- uncontrollable crying?
- brooding about the past?
- feelings of hopelessness?
- mood swings?
- deteriorating personal relationships?
- thoughts of suicide?

If you've been experiencing four or more of these symptoms, you may be suffering from depression. If you think this might be the case, keep in mind that depression is a treatable condition. With therapy or medication, or both, you can learn to manage it. To find a mental health practitioner, ask your doctor for a referral, call your local medical society, or ask a friend who may have had a similar experience.

USING THE MIND TO HEAL THE BODY

Unlike other organs in the body, the skin is always exposed to the ever changing world. It responds appropriately and immediately to touch, temperature, and emotion. Fear causes the skin's blood vessels to constrict, and your face becomes pale. Embarrassment causes the skin to flush with increased blood flow. Your health, both physical and mental, is displayed where everyone can see. To orchestrate this complex behavior, the skin has billions of nerve endings just waiting to shoot a message to the brain. In response to the skin's messages, the brain sends back sensations of fear, happiness, pain, or itch.

Just as negative emotions can make eczema worse, positive emotions can make it better. It is impossible to overemphasize the link between the emotions and the severity of eczema. If you have been ignoring this aspect, take a look at the following list of questions. They may help you make the connection between your moods and your eczema.

- ☐ Does your eczema fluctuate with your emotions?
- ☐ Do medically proven treatments not work for you?
- ☐ Are treatments only temporarily effective?
- ☐ Is your skin condition more stubborn than your doctor expects?

- ☐ Does your eczema change with important events, such as vacations, family gatherings, and promotions?
- ☐ Do you suppress your emotions?
- ☐ Are you highly distressed about your eczema?
- ☐ Are others surprised at your lack of distress?
- ☐ Do you hurt or pick at your skin?
- ☐ Do you feel overly dependent on your dermatologist?
- ☐ Do you feel overly angry with your dermatologist?
- ☐ Do others notice your skin improving before you do?
- ☐ Is it hard for you to acknowledge when your skin has improved?

If you answered "Yes" to most of the questions, then your emotions may have more control over your eczema than you do. To explore this further, start an eczema diary, marking down your feelings and the extent of your eczema. Learn which emotions make your eczema worse and which help it.

Laughter

Laughter is good medicine. It releases endorphins, the chemicals that elevate mood, lower blood pressure, and reduce stress. Endorphins are natural painkillers and itch relievers. While humor is a good way to cope with many of life's problems, it is especially helpful for eczema.

Sharing

Share your experiences with someone else suffering from eczema. No one understands what you're going through as well as a comrade in arms. Contact the National Eczema Association for Science and Education (see page 228 for the address) for an eczema support group near you. Your dermatologist may be willing to help you contact individuals with eczema who have designated an interest in meeting others who share their condition. Talking with someone who knows, understands, and listens to what you're going through can be a terrific relief. I can almost guarantee that you'll see an immediate improvement in your eczema just from knowing you're not alone.

Counseling

Psychological counseling by a mental health professional is an excellent way to learn to manage the emotional impact of eczema. Here's how it can help:

- It can help you see which difficulties are due to eczema and which aren't.
- It can help address your family's concerns. Your doctor should recognize that the person with eczema suffers, but so does his or her family.
- You can learn to be more consistent with your treatment. Many people with eczema suffer needlessly because they don't follow the course of treatment prescribed by their doctor. Through counseling, you can learn the root causes of your resistance.
- You can learn stress management techniques to reduce the psychological impact of eczema.
- You will learn to better communicate your needs to yourself, your family, your friends, and health care professionals.

If your doctor suggests counseling, don't be upset. He or she doesn't think you're crazy. A counselor will be one of the few doctors who understands how difficult it is to live with eczema.

YOUR FAMILY AND YOUR EMOTIONS

Poor communication can lead to misunderstanding. While most people know this on an intellectual level, it can be very difficult to change ingrained habits when it comes to talking with other people about eczema. This is doubly difficult with emotionally charged intimate relationships.

If one partner is suffering but doesn't explain what is bothering him or her, the other partner feels left out. If, on the other hand, the afflicted partner expresses all of his or her emotions, but doesn't receive the needed or expected response, he or she feels abandoned. If you have been either the stoic or the bereft, take charge. It's never too late to start communicating.

There are some basic ground rules that can help establish the type of atmosphere in which the needs of the person with eczema and family members can be met. To start, no one can help you without knowing your needs. Don't expect people to be able to read your mind; let them know what you're going through. If you need rest, express it in ways that your partner or family will understand. Try to avoid sounding angry, as if you're accusing them of something. For instance, you might say, "I'm not feeling well right now, and even making supper seems overwhelming. I'd appreciate as much help as you can give me." Or, "My rash is acting up, and I'm feeling uncomfortable and itchy. I'm sorry, I'll have to stay home, but I'd be very interested in hearing how it went." This kind of communication lets the other person know what the problem is, how it makes you feel, and the ways in which he or she can help you.

Try to be as kind toward yourself as you would like others to be toward you. It is not uncommon for people who have enjoyed good health to feel angry at themselves when an illness prevents them from doing the things they once could. Now is the time for you to be as compassionate and patient with yourself as you have been with your children, your partner, and others whom you have helped in times of trouble.

For family members of a person with eczema, remember that illness—particularly if it involves discomfort, pain, and anxiety—can affect the personality of the person who suffers from it. Even someone who is ordinarily upbeat and resilient can feel so uncomfortable and demoralized that the optimism you normally expect vanishes. Learn as much as possible about your loved one's condition, not only for your own sake but so you can be a valuable resource. There are many stories about family members who were the first to find out about helpful treatments or became important advocates for their loved ones because they had actively done their research.

Instead of waiting to be asked to help, volunteer to do the small things that let your loved one know you empathize with her or his discomfort. Prop up the pillows, make a cup of tea, buy a small gift—whatever you know the person will appreciate. Ask how your loved one feels. You may not be able to cure the physical condition, but your listening will keep your loved one from feeling alone in his or her suffering.

Talking to Your Children

Explaining your condition to children can be a challenge. For many children, a parent's illness is burdensome. Sometimes kids are called upon to sacrifice their normal activities to help at home. In other cases, children are kept in the dark because parents want to spare them worry. Either situation can cause resentment and guilt. It's a good idea to discuss your concerns openly with your children. Even very young children sense when there is a problem in the family. It's better to bring the problem out in the open, before your children imagine an explanation that is worse than the reality.

• • •

Combining a positive mental approach to eczema with a good home care routine will go far in keeping you eczema-free. A positive attitude will make you feel better, minimize your eczema flares, and make it easy for those around you to pitch in and help.

PART THREE
For Parents of Children with Eczema

Chapter Eleven

CARING FOR YOUR CHILD

Relief for itchy children is a vital issue for parents. A miserable child can traumatize families and actually harm the health of the suffering child. The solution to the misery is simple: parental education. Research has proven that the single most important tool for the control of eczema symptoms in children is *accurate* parental education about the disorder and about home care for their child.

Unfortunately, doctors rarely have time to explain details to parents. The result is that much of the advice about eczema floating around is a combination of anecdotal stories and ancient myths. Your child's pediatrician or a dermatologist is the only practitioner with correct medical information. The National Eczema Association for Science and Education is a respected American organization that provides excellent educational materials and contact information for support in your area. Avoid any group or practitioner who promises a miracle cure. There is none.

Caring for a child with eczema is stressful. Adding to the day-to-day issues is the guilt many parents carry that they have somehow done something to damage their child. Parents pass on genetic material to their offspring. If one or both parents have the defective genes that make their child susceptible to eczema, it doesn't mean the child will inevitably develop the disorder. The catalyst for the appearance of the symptoms is the child's environment.

Ironically, Western standards of cleanliness probably encourage the appearance of eczema. A too-clean nursery eliminates germs and pollens so the baby's immune system doesn't have a chance to build resistance to common environmental triggers. Later, when the child is exposed to the environment, his or her immune system doesn't react normally.

A child reared on a farm who plays in the dirt with other children and farm animals will probably not develop eczema regardless of the genes he or she carries. Once the child has developed eczema, an even higher standard of cleanliness is needed to keep the child from having flares. See the chapter on home care for tips on creating an eczema-free environment.

Parents of children with eczema should know these three important facts:

- Eczema is not caused by something your child ate.
- Eczema is not caused by something you did to your child.
- Eczema is not an allergy; it's an immune disorder.

ECZEMA AND INFANTS

While the term *eczema* is used for this disorder, eczema is technically only the visible rash created by scratching. Newborns don't have the motor skill to identify where they itch or the motor control to use their hands to scratch. Without the ability to scratch, infants with eczema will be miserable with itching. They cry, fuss, and wiggle in their cribs. You know something is wrong, but if the child doesn't have any visible signs—like a rash—to give you a clue to the problem, it's almost impossible to know how to relieve your baby's discomfort.

Even though they lack motor skills, babies are not completely helpless. Tiny babies can reach their faces with fists and tongues. Squirming against bedding can cause a rash on their faces. Some babies suffer such a frenzy of itchy restlessness that their constant wiggling can raise a rash all over their bodies. If you have a family history of eczema and an inconsolable baby, there's a strong possibility that your child is suffering from itching. It would probably be a good idea to ask your pediatrician for a referral to a dermatologist.

Eczema affects different parts of the body, depending upon age. In infants, the rash typically appears first on the face or scalp, since the skin is not covered and the baby can rub against bedding. However, that doesn't mean the child doesn't itch in other places. For the first line of defense, try this to keep your baby comfortable:

- Let the baby soak in lukewarm, not hot, water for at least 15 minutes. This will do two things: 1) While the baby is in the bath, he or she will not itch. 2) The water will be absorbed, which moisturizes the baby's skin.
- When you take the baby out of the bath, pat, don't rub, the water from the skin. Slather petroleum jelly on the child's body and face within *3 minutes* of removing him or her from the water. Be careful when handling your slippery baby.

- Don't dress or wrap the baby in wool. Wool fibers have tiny spikes that irritate eczema skin.
- Heat and perspiration are the two major causes of discomfort for anyone with eczema. This means keeping your babies and small children as cool as possible. Parents have a tendency to overdress babies. While mom and dad are walking around in shorts and T-shirts, their baby is often bundled up in layers of clothing and blankets. Babies and small children have a more efficient metabolism than adults, which means they need less clothing, not more, than you. If you are wearing lightweight clothing, so should your baby.
- Even small children can benefit from massage. Twenty minutes each day can visibly improve your child's mood and eczema. It also helps parents to relax.
- Put damp pajamas on your baby. This will keep the skin cool and moist, which reduces itching. Put dry pajamas over the wet ones to keep sheets dry.

Diaper Rash

Diaper rash is often mistaken for eczema in babies who have eczema elsewhere on their bodies. Diaper rash is usually caused by the friction of the diaper rubbing against skin or by the high acid content of the baby's stool. Urine doesn't cause diaper rash. All infants who wear diapers get diaper rash at some point, but it isn't more common with infants who have eczema.

CARING FOR TODDLERS

Toddlers can scratch their itchy skin. If the itch isn't suppressed, the child can fall into the itch-scratch-itch cycle, which can escalate into serious episodes. Intense scratching can also permanently damage their skin. In toddlers, the rash is often concentrated on knees and the inner part of the arm at the elbow, as well as the face and scalp. Pay particular attention to these areas when you are applying creams or moisturizers.

Teaching your child good home care should start as soon as possible. Toddlers can let you know where they itch even if they can't talk. Ask your child to point to where it itches. Starting some habits early makes them easier to accept as children get older.

- Teach your toddler to wear gloves during activities that can irritate skin. Gloves over topical medications can heal hands while they sleep.
- You might be able to teach a very young child to reach for a moisturizer like petroleum jelly when itching starts rather than scratching. Keep plenty of moisturizer in easy-to-use containers within reach of your child.

CARING FOR OLDER CHILDREN

Eczema tends to affect the skin over the joints in older children. The skin in this area may crack and bleed when arms and legs are flexed or extended if not cared for properly. A school-age child can be actively involved in his or her own care. You and your child need to be aware of the triggers that bring on flares and be prepared to manage them before they get out of control. Chapter 5 lists the most common causes of flares; however, there may be things that bother your child that are not mentioned. Know your child, and know what to watch out for. With experience, education, and cooperation, you and your child can create an itch-free environment (see chapter 8 for specific information). Don't underestimate the intelligence and capability of your child. Sharing responsibility with your child will create the best possible atmosphere for controlling itching.

First Aid

Children with eczema are at greater risk for skin infections. Regardless of the age of your child, check his or her skin daily for the following conditions:

Scratch Marks

- If they are shallow and few, keep track of them. Make sure they don't get infected, and be more attentive to the home care regimen.
- If the scratches are extensive and widespread, it's a sign that the child's eczema is significantly worse. Either you need to use prescription medication that you already have at home or you may need to call your doctor.

Infected Areas

- For infected areas, use antibacterial cleansers and topical antibiotics—either over-the-counter products or a prescription your doctor has given to you.
- If the infection doesn't get better or is widespread, or if your child has symptoms like chills, malaise, or fever, call your doctor.

Crusting

- Crusting can be the result of scratching eczema so hard and deeply that the scratching causes bleeding. In this case, intensify eczema treatment and use techniques to reduce scratching, such as antihistamines, nail trimming, bandages, and psychological relaxation techniques.

- If the crust is yellow or green, it might be infected. In that case, follow the aforementioned directions for infections.

Discolored Skin

- Red skin may indicate an eczema flare or an infection. If it doesn't respond to standard eczema treatment, call your doctor.
- If the discolored skin is yellow or green, it's probably infected. If your doctor has already given you medication and instructions for treating infections, then treat it at home. If it doesn't improve, call your doctor.
- If the discolored skin is light or dark, it may be eczema and require eczema therapy, or it may be a fungal infection and require antifungal treatment. Try an over-the-counter antifungal treatment first. If that's not successful, call your doctor.

Regardless of cause, if these conditions get progressively worse or haven't cleared within two weeks, call your child's doctor.

General Good Health

Children with eczema need to develop healthy habits early. If the following steps are taken, you'll be able to control infection:

- Keep stress to a minimum. Stress can trigger flares and lower immune system effectiveness. (See chapter 12 for tips on managing stress.)
- Be sure your child gets adequate sleep. Kids with eczema consistently get less sleep than other children. Tips for helping your child sleep follow on page 151.

Children with eczema are more likely to get skin infections and are more susceptible to childhood illnesses. When they do get infections, they are harder to control than in those without the disorder. The following simple suggestions will keep catching other people's germs to a minimum:

- Avoid anyone who is ill. Some germs are spread by breathing them.
- Wash hands after contact with public surfaces. While breathing in germs from sick people can spread disease, the most common way to be infected is by touching a surface covered with viruses or bacteria, then touching the eyes or mouth.
- Don't share towels. They are a breeding ground for many different unsavory life forms.
- Don't share eating utensils or drinking vessels. Contact is the best way to pick up other people's germs.
- Avoid drafts of cold air. Changes in air temperature cause congestion in airways and passages. When nasal passages, ear passages, and airways become congested, they are less able to flush out bacteria and viruses.

SUGGESTIONS FOR HELPING ITCHY KIDS

To stop an itch attack, try one of the following:

- Give your child an oatmeal bath in lukewarm water. Soak for at least 20 minutes, but not more than 30 minutes. Cover the skin thoroughly with the thickest cream your child can tolerate within 3 minutes of leaving the bath.

- Refrigerate any prescription medication or moisturizer. This will stop itching faster than room-temperature creams. For trips away from home, use a cooler.
- Make sure your child's skin is covered with an emollient like petroleum jelly before he or she goes swimming.
- Cover your child's face and hands with an emollient like petroleum jelly before he or she goes out in cold weather.
- Babies' hands and cheeks should be coated before meals so that foods and beverages don't irritate their skin.
- Have your child wear loose-fitting, comfortable clothes made of cotton or any other smooth-fiber fabric.
- When you purchase new clothing or bedding, wash it before your child uses it. Dyes, preservatives, and irritants on new fabric can leach onto the skin and cause itching.
- Keep your child's fingernails trimmed.
- Have your child wear cotton gloves at night. Knee-high socks are sometimes better because they don't fall off as easily.
- Keep your child's hands busy during the day. Idle hands will often find occupation in scratching. Try worry beads, hand-size squeeze balls, or hand toys.
- Try over-the-counter antihistamines. If oral antihistamines make your child drowsy, try a topical cream. Benadryl cream is often effective but does contain allergens that can cause an allergic reaction if overused, even in those without eczema. Ask your doctor if a prescription cream called Zonalon might help your child. Zonalon doesn't contain allergens.

For some children with eczema, scratching may become an obsessive habit. The child may be unconscious of scratching until he or she causes excessive pain or bleeding. It's important to help your child control the impulse to scratch. By observation and conversation, determine your child's itch pattern. A common but often not recognized cause is the friction of clothing on skin when your child changes. Another time to watch is when your child's attention is taken away from an engrossing activity, like watching TV or playing video games. Forgotten itching may suddenly demand a good scratch.

To help your child help him- or herself, be sure he or she is fully informed about the risks of scratching and the damage it can do. Have moisturizers and any other equipment readily available for quick access to relief. Teach your child how to use everything. There are alternatives to scratching that you can teach your child, like clenching the fists or lightly slapping the itchy skin. When you see your child scratching, start treatment. Try not to demand that your child stop scratching. This will only increase anxiety and stress for both of you. Help your child keep track of how often he or she scratches by keeping a diary. Go over it with him or her and discuss how bad the itching was and how the child managed it.

For those times when the child was really uncomfortable but managed to control the urge to itch, offer a reward. The reward needs to be appropriate to the child's interest. Rewards should also be consistent. If you promise your child a small gift, be sure to follow through. Disappointment will not help your child. Some parents have made a star or sticker chart, letting their child add a star or sticker each time he or she successfully conquers the urge to scratch.

SCHOOL ISSUES

Kids with a visible rash are often self-conscious about it. They either don't get involved in activities or find themselves excluded. Being ostracized makes children more likely to try drugs and alcohol or to join other outcasts in antisocial behavior. As a parent, you'll need to have good communication with your child from an early age.

This communication needs to be open enough for your child to tell you if he or she feels left out or embarrassed. If so, you'll need to educate your child's teachers and coaches about eczema. Only when the responsible parties at school understand eczema and educate your child's peers will there be a safe and caring environment for your child to participate fully in all school activities.

If you start with your child's elementary school, you'll probably be able to avert problems during the junior high and high school years. Don't wait until junior high school to talk to your child about drugs, alcohol, and cigarettes. Drugs and alcohol make eczema worse. Make sure that your child understands the additional hazards of these substances for eczema.

It isn't just illegal substances that are unhealthy for children with eczema. Clay, glue, and chalk dust may trigger flares. Makeup, perfume, and artificial nails can also cause problems. Cheap makeup contains sharp particles that can damage skin. Perfumes contain irritating chemicals, and artificial nails harbor fungus. Clothing made from plastic, rubber, leather, or wool shouldn't be worn by kids with eczema.

Dealing with Your Child's School

If your child has a difficult case of eczema, with frequent flares and a visible rash, you'll want to make sure the school employees understand how to help your child, both with teasing and with discomfort. Start with the school nurse. In large schools, he or she can provide medical care and make sure the staff understands your child's needs. In a smaller school, you might need to speak to the principal and ask for the best way to get emergency care for your child as well as get the information to the right people. If your child is active in sports, make sure the coach is aware of special needs, such as proper skin care and prevention of overheating.

Request that eczema education be included in the school health agenda. This will ensure that teachers and students will be aware of the condition. You can even invite your doctor to give a talk at your child's school. Ask what the school's policy is on teasing and harassment. If you're not satisfied, you might want to speak to the principal.

Several excellent organizations provide extensive information online or will send you pamphlets upon request:

- American Academy of Dermatology, www.aad.org.
- Society for Pediatric Dermatology, www.pedsderm.net.
- National Eczema Association for Science and Education, www.nationaleczema.org.

If you feel that in spite of your best efforts your child is suffering at school, you might want to consider the possibility of changing to a school where the atmosphere is healthier and more accepting.

Visiting Other Children's Homes

No matter how careful you are to prevent flares at home, if your child visits a place not geared for those with eczema, he or she may be overwhelmed by flare triggers. Before sending your child off to a friend's house, camp, or even school, make up an eczema travel kit that your child can take along. The kit should contain the following:

- ☐ **Medications,** such as steroid cream for flares.
- ☐ **Cleansers.** It's best that your child not use regular soaps or products that can irritate the skin.
- ☐ **Moisturizers.** This should be either a travel-size variety of the regular product or a larger size, depending upon the length of the stay.
- ☐ **Personal care items.** This would include products made especially for sensitive skin.
- ☐ For overnight stays, pack **linens, pillows, and blankets** that you are sure your child doesn't react to.
- ☐ Include **instructions on eczema care** for the responsible adults just in case your child suffers an unexpected flare.
- ☐ **Emergency contact information** should include the parents' phone number and the number of the child's doctor.

Make sure hosts are aware of your child's eczema and special needs. The best way is to call in advance and explain your child's condition. Find out if there are particular triggers at the place your child will be staying and add necessary items to the kit. If you feel that your child won't be safe, offer to host the sleepover at your house.

HELPING YOUR CHILD TO SLEEP

Children with eczema get less sleep than children who don't for a very obvious reason: Itching keeps them from relaxing enough to fall asleep. Itching attacks can also flare in the middle of the night, waking the child and everyone else in the house.

Lack of sleep is serious. Tired children don't learn as well as those who get a good night's sleep. Sleep deprivation can make a child cranky and anxious. Over the long term, it can affect the child's general health. Lack of sleep for the child's parents is just as serious. Tired parents lose patience with their fussy child, creating stress—which makes the child's eczema worse. The first thing is to reduce tension and stress in the family. Explore meditation and relaxation techniques. To help your child sleep better, be sure you are doing everything possible to keep itching under control during the day. Include an itch check at bedtime to see that all medications and moisturizers are doing their jobs. Remember that clear skin can itch, so if your child complains of itching but you don't see a rash, treat the area just as aggressively as you would if the skin were broken. Don't forget to check your child's scalp. Hair hides the rash of eczema very well, particularly in children with thick hair. The only clue may be mild dandruff. When you inspect closely, you may see telltale signs of eczema or even scrapes and scratches to indicate nocturnal digging. Scalp preparations for eczema are different from skin preparations. Your doctor may prescribe medication especially for scalps.

Baths about an hour before bedtime followed by emollients and medications (if needed) can reduce itching. Your child's skin will be cool and comfortable at bedtime. Apply creams to your child's skin at least 20 minutes before bedtime to give them time to be absorbed. If you apply them too close to bedtime, the stickiness may be irritating.

If your child isn't really tired, it will be harder for him or her to fall asleep. Most scratching tends to occur between getting into bed and drifting off to sleep. Put your drowsy child in a bed provided with bedding made from comfortable, natural fabrics like cotton. Scratchy fabrics or wool will only make itching worse at night. If your child wears pajamas or a nightgown to bed, be sure it's made of a loose, comfortable fabric, preferably cotton. To minimize damage to the skin at night, put your child to bed in one-piece pajamas. Wrap especially itchy places with medicated or wet bandages over ointment. You can also rub ointment on the rash and put damp pajamas next to the skin with dry pajamas on top.

If your child is too warm, he or she will itch more. If you live in a high-pollution or high-dust area, use window filters to keep your child's room free of irritants. If there is a heat source or a radiator in the room, make sure your child's bed is not right next to it. Direct heat can make the bed too warm as well as dry out exposed skin, leading to worse itching. Gentle fans or air-conditioning in the summer can help keep the bedroom cool.

Keep pets out of your child's bedroom to maintain a mite-, dander-, and dust-free haven in which to sleep. If the family dog enters your child's bedroom to sniff around just once, a whole week of dust and mite reduction measures is undone. Don't let cigarette or cigar smoke get into the bedroom. Smoke contains particulate matter that can irritate the skin directly. It also irritates the airways; this reduces your child's comfort and makes it harder for him or her to get sleep.

Once a child falls asleep, chances are good that he or she will sleep throughout the night. Only if the eczema is severe or if your child is very uncomfortable will he or she wake up repeatedly. That's why getting your child to sleep in the first place is crucial for both of you.

Bedtime rituals help all children but are especially helpful for those with eczema. If you have trouble getting your child in the proper frame of mind for sleep, try some of the following suggestions:

- Bedtime stories are always good.
- Unless your child objects to your voice, sing a lullaby.
- Let your child fall asleep on your lap before putting him or her to bed.
- Snuggle the child in the car and let the vibrations of the motor work their magic.
- If possible, eliminate naps so your child will be sleepier at night.
- Eliminate all forms of caffeine, such as those found in soft drinks and chocolates.
- Let your child stay up until he or she is really tired.

In difficult times, you might consider medications that can help your child sleep. It's a good idea to talk to your child's doctor about a prescription sleeping aid. Over-the-counter antihistamine tablets have been safely used for eczema. They work in two ways: First, by making your child drowsy, they send him or her off to sleep quickly. You'll have to manage the dose carefully so your child is not groggy the next day. Second, by inhibiting histamine, one of the body's natural chemicals responsible for the itch sensation, antihistamines reduce itching. Use antihistamines for up to a week to break the cycle of scratching. It's a good idea to give antihistamines to your child about an hour before bedtime so they have a chance to work. Some children do better sleeping with their parents. If it works, do it; if not, don't. You've probably already come up with some creative ideas on your own.

Crying and Scratching Spells at Night

It's three in the morning and your child is wailing. This is a common occurrence in families dealing with eczema. Here are some suggestions to get your child comfortable and back to sleep:

- Your presence alone is comforting to your child.
- Ask where the itch is and apply cream to those areas.
- If the itching is generalized, apply the cream all over in a gentle massage until your child falls asleep.
- If your child's scratching is damaging the skin, cover it up with a soft, self-sticking bandage like Coban or Kerlix.
- If your child balks at bandages or creams, offer a reward for cooperation.
- Try to anticipate nighttime flares by putting cream and bandages on your child before he or she goes to bed. Treating a sleepy, crying child is hard on everyone.

Finally, children sleep poorly for a number of reasons. If your child is cranky and not sleeping properly, and you've done all you can to address eczema, consider other possibilities, like nightmares. If he or she has asthma or rhinitis, is breathing the issue? Has your child been hurt or injured and now can't find a comfortable sleeping position? As the parent of an eczema child, you need to be attentive to eczema, but don't automatically rule out other possibilities.

Childhood Illnesses

Smallpox

Those with eczema should never be given the smallpox vaccine. Because of the damaged skin barrier, smallpox can take hold and either kill the child or leave him or her terribly and permanently scarred.

Chicken Pox

If your child is using a steroid cream or taking a steroid medication for eczema or diseases associated with eczema like asthma, you need to be careful about chicken pox. If your child has been exposed to it or developed a case of chicken pox, see your doctor immediately. The disease can be quite dangerous for someone on steroids. Your doctor will need to give your child an antibody boost or antiviral medication to deal with the infection.

Viruses

All kids get colds, flu, and viral infections like mumps and measles. At this time, there is no evidence that childhood viruses affect eczema. They neither exacerbate nor help cure the condition.

Infections

Infections caused by bacteria, viruses, or fungi can make your child's eczema worse or slow down healing. If you have been actively treating eczema for two weeks and it gets progressively worse or doesn't improve, see your doctor.

Bacterial Infections of the Skin

The best defense here is to be sure the skin remains moist and supple. Dry skin is a welcome home for staphylococcus. If your child uses a good emollient cream at home daily and regularly, staphylococcus shouldn't take hold. However, if your child has frequent recurrences of infected eczema, talk to your doctor about prevention.

Viral Infections of the Skin

The virus responsible for cold sores is herpes simplex. It usually affects the face, especially the lips. If your child gets cold sores, you'll need antiviral medication prescribed by your child's doctor. If you yourself have cold sores, be careful not to spread them to your child through touch (if not on the face) or kissing (if on the face).

Molluscum contagiosum, caused by a poxvirus, is another common viral infection found on the skin of eczema patients. Red or skin-colored bumps appear primarily in the rash area, but can pop up anywhere on the body. The bumps range in size from a pinpoint to that of a lentil. Scratching spreads the virus from one part of the body to another. While it's unusual for it to spread from person to person, it's still a good idea not to share towels, intimate clothing, or bedding. This virus won't go away by itself, so see a doctor if you or your child develop suspicious bumps on the skin. Warts are also common in eczema. Treat them with over-the-counter remedies or see your doctor.

USING STEROIDS

Thanks to the media uproar over steroid abuse by athletes, some parents are reluctant to give them to their child. However, the steroids abused in the sports world are anabolic steroids taken orally and are completely different from the steroid creams prescribed for eczema.

Steroids don't cure eczema, but they work wonderfully well in suppressing flares if used according to a doctor's instructions. However, if they aren't used properly, steroids can make eczema worse, damage skin, and, in extreme cases, damage internal organs. Teaching parents the proper use of steroids is the single most important safety measure for using them. While parental education is key, be sure the information you get is from a doctor well trained in the use of steroids. Even though you trust your pediatrician and primary care doctor, dermatologists are the best source for exact instructions on using steroids.

As helpful as steroids are for eczema, they should be used only as an adjunct to rigorous home care. Steroids can't do the job alone. I tell my patients to use medications for up to two weeks, followed by a two-week break. During the break, use moisturizers only.

Steroids vary in potency. Low-potency steroids are prescribed for sensitive skin areas, such as the face, armpits, and genitals. Higher-potency steroids are prescribed for thicker skin, like the palms, soles, and scalp. For all areas, use the lowest potency that controls your child's eczema.

For moisturizing, most doctors prefer that their patients use an ointment over a cream. The thicker ointments have longer staying power and penetrate the skin better for a longer time than creams. But ointments are thick and greasy and hard to apply. Children often object to the stickiness, so parents find creams easier to use. Creams don't suppress itching quite as well as ointments except in cases of weeping eczema, when a cream is preferred.

Your doctor will have a plan for you to deal with your flare. I normally recommend a few days of potent steroid medication followed by a few weeks of weekend-only potent steroid medication. Some practitioners recommend twice daily steroid treatment for one or two weeks, followed by a holiday period of one to two weeks. On treatment and nontreatment days, emollients should be used. Other practitioners use potent steroid medication for a few days and follow this with an ointment for a few days, followed by a very mild steroid preparation for longer periods.

Topical Immunomodulators

TIMs are a new family of steroid-free drugs that have revolutionized eczema therapy. They are safer than steroids and approved for use in infants. Regular use of TIMs has been shown to make flares easier to treat or even prevent them altogether. TIMs are an effective and safe substitute for steroids. The only problem reported is that there is sometimes a "burning" sensation when they are applied. This can be prevented by keeping TIMs in the refrigerator. Examples of TIMs are Elidel (pimecrolimus) and Protopic (tacrolimus).

FOR YOU, THE PARENTS

Remember that although there is no cure for eczema at this time, most children grow out of it. The condition can be controlled in a majority of cases with simple treatment. You should discuss your child's eczema with your doctor rather than experiment yourself. Here are some general pointers to help keep you healthy and sane while dealing with your child's eczema:

Take care of yourself. You're of no use to your child if you're tired and stressed. Parents often sacrifice their own health and their own needs to take care of their children. With eczema, you need all the patience, stamina, and understanding you can muster to take care of your child, especially if your child has severe eczema. You'll also need to reinforce daily lessons so that your child can treat him- or herself independently as soon as possible. If you're not feeling your best, you won't be able to give your best.

Learn everything you can about eczema. Check out the resources listed in the appendix for additional help. When you become part of the larger eczema community, you'll find support from other families.

Find a good doctor to treat your child's eczema. While most pediatricians can treat mild eczema, it's still a good idea to consult a dermatologist. If your child has special needs, be sure that your child's dermatologist has access to advanced treatment techniques. Visit the dermatologist to be sure you are comfortable with your relationship. You're likely to be working together for quite some time, and it's important that your philosophies mesh.

Don't stop learning. Research in eczema is progressing at a rapid rate. We are learning more about causes and treatments daily. Follow health news in newspapers, magazines, TV, and the Internet. Keep in touch with your support network for the latest ideas on care. Ask your doctor at each visit if new treatments are in use. You'll be surprised how often new information turns up. Your child's comfort is directly related to how well you understand eczema.

Chapter Twelve

PSYCHOLOGICAL IMPACT

No child wants to live with the miserable discomfort of eczema. Eczema children are engaged in a solitary battle against an unseen enemy that has invaded their bodies. They feel trapped in their own skins. Some children describe the itching as being possessed by an evil spirit. Some have wished for an out-of-body experience so they could get away from their burning skin.

Adding to the physical misery is the unpredictable nature of eczema. Even when the itching has stopped, the child anxiously and fearfully waits for the next attack. While there's no question that eczema is a physiological disorder of the skin's immune system, it should come as no surprise that the more severe the eczema, the greater the emotional distress of the sufferer and the sufferer's family. It's important to understand what your child is suffering, but it's also important to know that there's a lot you can do about it. Every member of the family is affected when one child has eczema. In this chapter, I'll discuss the psychological issues faced by parents, siblings, and the eczema child. Most important are suggestions for managing a seemingly unmanageable problem.

CHILDREN WITH ECZEMA

Difficulties for children with eczema start early. One of the most unfortunate consequences of newborn eczema is that it can have a profound impact on mother-baby bonding. The close and intimate touch that is so essential to this relationship can be perceived by the baby as an itchy sensation. Rather than cuddling up to the mother, the baby with eczema may cry and struggle to get away from the discomfort.

Children with eczema try constantly to stop themselves from scratching. They tuck their hands under their arms. They feign paralysis. The harder they try, the harder it is to resist the urge. They try nondamaging ways to scratch. They rub instead of dig. They pinch themselves. They ration their scratching, telling themselves to scratch only their legs when in fact their whole body is on fire.

It's tempting to yell at them to stop scratching. You can't feel it, and sometimes you suspect they're doing it just to get your attention. This isn't true. Children with eczema scratch when they are alone and there's no one around to pay attention to them. If you tell a child that the scratching is all in his or her head, you are suggesting that it's the child's fault, the implication being that if the child wanted to stop itching, he or she could. This is an unfair case of blaming the victim. On the other hand, it's not uncommon for a suffering child to take advantage of the situation. The child gets more attention or less punishment for bad behavior when he or she plays the eczema card.

Eczema can't be wished away, and psychotherapy can't cure eczema. But easing stress helps everyone. Among my patients, the psychological effects of eczema are fairly consistent. Kids with eczema worry all the time about almost everything. They are aware they are the center of much of their family's conflict. When a new treatment doesn't work, they think it's their fault. They are anxious about going to school for fear of an unexpected flare or the taunts of the classmates. This results in crying spells and stomachaches. They have trouble sleeping, not just because of the itching, but also because of the worry. As stressful as their lives are, children with eczema rarely cause disruptions at school. This stress is more likely to come out in a flare than in bad behavior.

Studies have shown that kids with eczema have twice the emotional difficulties of kids without eczema. Among children with moderate eczema, 53 percent have some evidence of psychological problems. Among kids with severe eczema, the figure is closer to 80 percent. On the scale used to measure this impact—the Rutter scale of psychological disturbance—other diseases had a far lower impact on the psychological well-being of children.

For example, 38 percent of children with leukemia have emotional problems. Only kids with hemiplegia—a form of paralysis—exhibited the same degree of psychological disturbances, about 55 percent. Children with *moderate* eczema and children with paralysis have equivalent emotional reactions. Imagine the emotional impact severe eczema can have on a child.

With eczema, it's the psychological component that's most devastating to kids. They've told me that they can play soccer and want to play, but they are afraid to or ashamed to. They want to be part of the group, but they feel left out. This feeling may be based on reality or may be based on the child's own perceptions. Either way, the child always feels like an outsider.

LOWERING THE ITCH THRESHOLD

Itching originates in the skin, but it's modified in the brain. Itching can be triggered by thinking about it. Ask people to not to think about how much the tip of their nose itches. Then tell them to not scratch their nose. Suddenly, their nose will start to itch and they feel an irresistible urge to scratch. This same mechanism affects children with eczema. All a parent has to do is demand that the child stop itching and the need to scratch intensifies.

Because of this psychological component of the intensity of itching, it's possible to teach a child how to raise or lower the itch threshold. Sometimes children discover this on their own, but most could use some help from their parents.

You can teach children to control the level of itching with imagery. Have the child sitting comfortably and with eyes closed. Tell him or her to imagine the itch as a flame. A mild itch may appear as a lighted match. Tell the child to gently blow out the match. Tell him or her that when the flame is gone, the itch will also be gone. A severe itch may be imagined as a raging bonfire. Children can come up with different ways of putting out the fire. They might imagine themselves as firefighters in full regalia with powerful water hoses.

Encourage your child to incorporate this type of imagery into his or her daily self-care regimen. Suggest that your child envision the application of creams or medication as magic potions that smother the itch. Or perhaps your child might visualize having hands with magic powers, able to quench flames just by touching or squeezing an itchy area instead of scratching it. If the whole body is itching, your child can imagine a cool day in the Arctic, with snow falling all over his or her body, soothing the flaming skin.

TEENAGERS

Adolescents with eczema have special needs. At a time when they want most of all to be like everyone else, they may not be able to wear popular fashions, are prevented from joining overnights because of a bad environment for eczema sufferers, or can't use trendy cosmetic products.

One common form of rebellion among teenagers with eczema is to refuse to continue with self-care. It's no surprise that they get tired of the constant vigilance and extra effort needed to keep their skin eczema-free. This is especially common among kids who haven't had a flare for a while and believe they've been cured. Most teens are aware of how important self-care is. They can see for themselves the consequences of ignoring it; however, sometimes they test their parents. If your teen stops self-care and raises a flare, will you take notice and step in? Or will you ignore the problem or lose your temper in frustration? It's important for parents to recognize these bids for attention. Show teens that you care about them.

There is no way to shield your child from social pressure to engage in self-destructive behavior. However, some basic information may help your child understand why certain substances are more harmful for him or her:

- Smoking causes eczema to flare.
- Alcohol causes flushing and warming of the skin, which triggers itching. Alcohol can also have dangerous interactions with antihistamines, particularly sedating antihista-

mines. The combination can reduce your child's level of awareness and make driving dangerous. In some cases, it can cause your child to lose consciousness.

- Tranquilizers have the same effect on your child's body as alcohol.
- Stimulants can make itching worse.
- Drug withdrawal can also make itching worse.

While there are no studies on whether or not drug use is more common among children with eczema, it is clear that children with eczema are more vulnerable to side effects.

School

As we all know, school can be a cruel place. Children isolate, ostracize, and mock anyone who is different, and the unsightly rash and constant scratching of eczema are sure to draw unwanted attention. The tactics of fellow students range from overt bullying to backbiting to cool isolation. This type of exclusion can occur on the playground, out of sight of any adult. It happens in the classroom right under the teacher's nose. Children with eczema may be embarrassed to tell their parents about it. To protect their feelings, they build an emotional shell that interferes with making close friends. These children often lack self-confidence, which adds to their isolation. They're often excluded by other children from play or sports and soon learn not to bother to try to join in.

This devastating rejection happens to children during a time when their sense of self is developing. Rejection by other children at an early age can have a lifelong negative effect on eczema sufferers. A study of preschool children with eczema found that they were shy, dependent, and fearful. They had 50 percent more behavioral problems than their eczema-free peers. Depression in children with eczema tends to rise with the severity of the disorder.

For all children, but especially for a child with eczema, an accepting atmosphere at school is essential. Bullying, exclusion from activities, and discrimination add to your child's burden. You can help by being involved in school affairs and making sure that your child's eczema is taken care of properly.

As a parent, you need to be aware of problems your child might be having at school. Rejection by peers often results in depression, which is very serious and not something a child should have to face alone. Talk to the school officials to see if something can be done to reduce rejection. If not, see if it's possible to change your child's school.

PARENTS

Guilt and Stress

Because accurate information about eczema is not easy to find, parents tend to blame themselves for causing their child's eczema. Parents who were careful with their diets during pregnancy and avoided alcohol and cigarettes will spend endless hours reexamining every bite, every drink, every chemical to which they were exposed, trying to identify the one thing they did that caused their child's eczema. Or perhaps one parent had eczema as a child and, since it had vanished long ago, never mentioned it to his or her spouse. The former eczema sufferer may feel guilty that he or she didn't look into possible hereditary conditions before getting pregnant. Parents blaming themselves or each other for their child's condition doesn't help and, in fact, adds even more stress to the health and stability of the marriage.

Eczema is not the result of children's psychological problems, nor is it caused by bad parenting. For too many years, every problem a child had was blamed on a cold or incompetent mother. The parents of any ill child will be less relaxed and more stressed than parents of a healthy child, regardless of which illness their child has. Eczema is especially difficult because it's not life-threatening and therefore not regarded as a serious problem by those who aren't affected by it.

Studies of parents of children with eczema have shown how serious their stress can be. When these parents were asked if they would have more children, many said they wouldn't. In other words, they are so emotionally drained from the child or children they already have that they wouldn't consider having any more.

The unpredictability of the disease undermines parents' confidence in their ability to care properly for their child. Lack of consistent results from treatments and confusion about eczema's cause result in their seeking alternative care. A 2003 study in the United Kingdom found that 46 percent of parents use alternative medicine to care for their children with eczema. Another 17 percent reported they intended to try alternative cures, despite the fact that only 14 percent believed they are more effective. The frustration parents experience is an indictment of the health care their children are receiving.

Parents of children with eczema seek help from doctors. Too often they're given a prescription and sent on their way. The doctor doesn't take the time to explain home care, and the parents don't know what to ask. There are ample statistics on how dissatisfied parents of children with eczema are with their doctors. Only 19 percent of the parents thought the treatments were "very effective." Almost 75 percent of the parents worried that the treatments doctors prescribed would have harmful side effects.

Doctors believed they were doing a better job: 44 percent

thought their treatments were very effective. This is more than a twofold disparity in the conception between doctors and parents of how useful doctors' treatments are. It clearly shows that medical management of eczema is handled very badly. Parents and patients don't get essential information on home care and use of medications. I don't blame parents for turning away from doctors to find relief for their children. I hope this book will give parents the help they so badly need.

Isolation

Parents of children with eczema feel isolated because they spend so much time taking care of their sick child. They have little time or energy left for socializing. Add to this the extra effort required to organize the skin care supplies needed for the child with eczema, and outings no longer seem appealing. Studies have shown that fewer mothers of children with eczema feel they have adequate social interaction and support compared with mothers of children without eczema. Maternal distress is even greater when she's home with a preschool child.

There is another form of isolation parents of children with eczema experience: the workplace. Almost two-thirds of mothers work. However, less than one-third of the mothers of children with eczema work. When working mothers quit to be at home with a child with eczema, they have lost an important part of their own identity. Parents who take time off from work because of a sick child are resented by co-workers. If absences are frequent, they can also miss out on promotions and raises. The loss of income can compound the stress of eczema.

Dealing with Anger

It should be no surprise that many parents are angry. They're angry at themselves, their spouse, their genes, and even their child. Anger is a scary emotion, one that is often suppressed but that will eventually erupt. Following are some suggestions for keeping peace at home.

Accept that neither you nor your spouse caused your child's eczema. Eczema is not your fault, your spouse's fault, or the fault of anyone in either family. It is not your child's fault. Tell your child that he or she is not to blame. Acknowledge to your child that he or she may be uncomfortable with itching, is worried about it, and is probably frightened by its consequences. Admit to yourself that your child certainly does not want it and in no way caused it.

Involve your child in your search for information. Discuss treatment options and try out suggestions together. When your child sees you taking an active role in learning about eczema and trying to conquer it, he or she will feel less alone. Educate your child. Children are proud of acquiring new skills, and a child who can take care of him- or herself will have more self-confidence. You will spend less time fretting over the child.

Insist that both parents share equally the burden of caring for this child. Sharing may not mean identical tasks for both parents. You may volunteer for daily baths, while your spouse makes sure the child's room is eczema-free. If you are a single parent, you will need help from friends, family, or, if possible, a paid outsider.

Treat your child fairly. Do not give him or her a break because of having eczema. It's important not to be overindulgent or overprotective. It's okay to reward the child to encourage good behavior, but the same system of rewards and punishments should apply to the other children for the same types of behaviors.

Do things as a family, involving everyone in activities so that neither the child with eczema nor other family members feel excluded. Find things that you can all do together. The beach is a particularly good choice, because salt water is very soothing to eczema skin and it's a great place for the whole family to get together. Participate in activities that involve you and your children. You may find group activities through your religious organization, the school, or local clubs. Participate in activities that keep you and your children active and involved with others. You'll be amazed how well this relieves stress. As you make friends, you'll also discover the many other families who are dealing with eczema.

Finally, take care of yourself. Accept that your life is stressful because you have a child with eczema. Find ways to manage your stress. Seek comfort in your faith. Take up a relaxing hobby or one that engages you and takes you out of your day-to-day mind-set. Talk with friends about your stress. Try relaxation techniques such as yoga or meditation.

Money

As if the psychological stress weren't bad enough, families are also burdened with financial stress. Between medical costs, hospital costs, and out-of-pocket expenses, the cost of caring for a child with eczema is greater than the cost of caring for a child with type 1 (juvenile) diabetes.

The costs rise depending upon the severity of the disease. Caring for someone with moderate eczema is three times as expensive as caring for someone with mild eczema. Taking care of someone with severe eczema is five times more expensive than caring for someone with a mild version.

The best way to keep costs down is to prevent flares in the first place. This reduces the need for treatment, medication, and hospitalization. Once a flare develops, treat it immediately and aggressively. If not treated quickly, a minor flare can develop into a serious, and costly, attack. Ask your pharmacist for generic medications when possible rather than buying proprietary drugs.

Buy skin care products by listed ingredients rather than brand name. More expensive doesn't always mean better quality. Ingredients to avoid are listed on pages 80–81. Recommended skin care products are listed in the Appendix.

Make sure your insurance policy covers eczema care. Check to see that it allows you to get access to specialists, treatment, and medications you need at the lowest cost possible.

Don't ignore the psychological aspects of eczema. Psychotherapy, hypnosis, and behavioral therapy make eczema more bearable and less severe. There's an up-front cost for these treatments, but once techniques are learned, they can be practiced for free in your own home. Join a group like the National Eczema Association to talk with others in your situation and learn tips on reducing costs.

SIBLINGS

Siblings of children with eczema suffer, too. All children have a limitless need for love and attention from their parents. In large families, especially when the children are close in age, there's fierce competition for parental attention. If one child wins the competition, the others feel they've lost out. Sisters and brothers get less attention because their parents are busy with the child with eczema. Eczema becomes the focal point around which family life is organized.

Sometimes parents express their guilt for their child's suffering through over indulgence. As a result, parents may be more generous with the child with eczema than good sense or good parenting dictates. This type of appeasement doesn't help anyone—neither the child nor the child's siblings.

Siblings show their resentment toward you and the child with eczema by acting out and behaving badly. If you discipline them harshly, this will make them further resent the sibling with eczema and convince them that you are in cahoots with the sick child. If there are several siblings who feel they get no support from their parents, they may form a clique that excludes the child with eczema. In their minds, the family is really two families: one consisting of the parents and the child with eczema, the other consisting of the unaffected siblings.

The first step to solving sibling jealousy is recognizing that it may be happening in your family. If so, you may find it comforting to know that this problem is common in families with a child with eczema. It doesn't mean you have a dysfunctional family. It means you have a problem that can be solved.

Talk to family members. Let the resentful siblings have their say. Acknowledge their unhappiness and discuss with them what would make them happier. If one parent is taking care of the child with eczema, make sure the other parent is sharing quality time with the other child(ren). Take every opportunity to tell each and every one of your children how special they are and how much you love them. Don't take sides in arguments. Try to be impartial in sibling disputes. Dole out praise and discipline equally and fairly. Praise your children for being good to one another. If this doesn't work or if the resentment is deep-seated, get outside help. Talk to eczema support groups for advice. Find a family therapist to help you get through this difficult problem.

If other relatives such as uncles, aunts, and grandparents also give preferred attention to the child with eczema, the unaffected siblings will feel even more isolated and resentful. Siblings suffer from jealousy, guilt, overprotectiveness, and even embarrassment for their sick brother or sister. If you need to, have private discussions with other members of your family and in-laws to make clear how much you value fair and equal treatment for each member of your family. Tell them how much you appreciate the extra interest they take in your child with eczema.

THERAPY

We know from studies that the emotional impact of eczema on children is as great as or greater than the physical impact. Even so, some of my patients and their parents will walk out of my office if I even hint that they should seek psychological help. I strongly recommend therapy for my patients with eczema and, sometimes, therapy for the entire family. The medical profession has done a poor job of explaining the physical and emotional aspects of the disease.

Treating the emotional aspects of eczema goes a long way toward helping children with their struggles. It has an overall positive impact on their self-esteem, on their interactions with family members and peers, and in their overall emotional development. For far less than the cost of medication, hospitalization, and office visits, proper attention to the psychology of eczema can vastly improve a child's quality of life.

If your doctor suggests you or your child get therapy, don't be offended or insulted. Know that your doctor recognizes the overall impact eczema has on your life. Be glad you have found a doctor who listens as well as hears.

The right therapist will teach you and your child the skills for managing the psychological aspects of eczema in a relatively short time. Work with your doctor and your insurance company to find ways in which this type of care can be covered. As newer studies demonstrate the benefit of therapy in the total management of eczema, you will have better data to support your claim. Your doctor may be able to help you petition for coverage. It may be clear that in the long run, your insurance company and you will save money by combining appropriate psychological techniques with medication to best manage your child's eczema. Your doctor may be affiliated with an institution that offers courses for coping with eczema. These may be available at reduced cost.

HOME STRESS REDUCTIONS

There are many ways to reduce the stress of eczema on your child with eczema and other members of your family:

- Take charge of your schedule by learning how to budget your time. Time is a commodity in short supply when a child has eczema. There are several excellent books on time management. I like *Manage Your Time* by Tim Hindle and *It's About Time!* by Linda Sapadin.
- Get a good stereo system. Music is such a potent drug that it has been banned in sporting events as a performance enhancer. It reduces fatigue and promotes a sense of well-being. Music means different things to different people. It can be the sound of waterfalls and waves, monks chanting, opera, classical music, or classic punk. Be sure one person's music doesn't invade another's comfort zone. Headphones would be a good idea in this case. Add music to household chores to dispel drudgery. Listen to your favorite music in the car when there's a traffic jam or kids squabbling in the backseat.
- After 2:00 p.m., don't take caffeine. Remember that colas, chocolates, teas, and some medications contain hidden caffeine. Don't let your child drink a big glass of any liquid before bedtime, to keep nighttime bathroom visits to a minimum.

- Keep your family active to reduce stress and improve the quality of sleep. As a family or individually, make sure everyone walks, jogs, bikes, or swims. Any activity is better than no activity.
- People who are in touch with their spirituality cope better with illness. Any religion or spiritual philosophy works.
- Attention to grooming and personal appearance elevates self-esteem. A tidy home is an eczema-free home.
- Laughter truly is excellent medicine. Studies have shown that a good belly laugh releases endorphins into the blood and therefore raises one's sense of well-being. Select humor that everyone in the family can enjoy. Stay away from put-down humor.

A united family is the best support a child with eczema can have. Thinking of the family as a team is crucial to dealing successfully with a child's eczema.

PART FOUR
Taking Control

Chapter Thirteen

TREATMENTS FOR ECZEMA

It's quite possible that your eczema will be very severe at some periods of your life and less so at others. If treatment strategies stop working, it may be necessary to try new ones. In addition to medical advice from your doctor, you'll probably hear lots of suggestions from friends on treatments that have worked for them. Many of these treatments are described in this chapter in terms of what they are and what we know about their efficacy. Few of the many eczema treatments have been studied rigorously. Some seem to work even though there's no evidence to support their use. To best manage your own care, you should know what doctors know about these different kinds of treatments. Some treatments your doctor might suggest won't be found in medical texts but are the result of years of experience with patients. Most of these treatments are never researched or written down because the doctors don't have time to do so.

Because each person has different needs, your treatment won't be identical to anyone else's. An appropriate course of treatment will balance cost, risks, and benefits. Ideally, your doctor will choose the treatment that is least expensive, least harmful, and easiest to follow.

Eczema treatments sometimes fail. The main reason is thought to be that patients either didn't follow their doctor's advice or didn't fully understand the instructions. Some patients believed a successful treatment meant the eczema would be cured. When flares erupted, they felt the treatment had failed and discontinued it. There is also a persistent but wrong belief that eczema is an allergy and if they avoid certain foods, the eczema will go away. Eczema is a chronic, genetic disorder. It will always be part of you and will always require some treatment.

The treatments described in this chapter are organized into four groups:

- Treatments supported by research
- Treatments with initial research results that seem encouraging
- Treatments that seem to work but require more research
- Treatments with no supporting research

Much of the following information was extracted from the *Cochrane Review,* produced by a public interest group that analyzes the quality of medical research and its results. You can find reports on recent research at www.cochrane.org.

TREATMENTS SUPPORTED BY RESEARCH

Cyclosporine

Cyclosporine is an immunomodulator, originally developed to prevent rejection of transplanted tissue. Dermatologists prescribe it to treat many different immune-mediated skin disorders, including eczema. Oral cyclosporine is toxic; however, it's very effective in reducing severe eczema symptoms. It also helps patients sleep and reduces the need for steroids. It's used only on a short-term basis because it's toxic and can lead to kidney failure and hypertension. Topical preparations are preferable because of its toxicity.

Psychological Therapy

Many different techniques are used to treat various aspects of eczema. Because the brain can modify somewhat the extent of a sufferer's discomfort, all show very good results. No one is preferable, nor are they mutually exclusive. Try several, and if they work, keep using them. Here are some approaches that have good results:

- Relaxation techniques
- Therapy that helps to manage the stressors that trigger flares
- Habit-reversal therapy to manage scratching
- Participation in support groups
- Psychological therapy that delves into the nature of eczema and its impact on the individual

Topical Steroids

Topical steroids are probably the most commonly prescribed and effective medication for eczema currently available.

They treat the symptoms very successfully but don't offer a permanent cure. Steroids have side effects, so it's important that you work closely with your doctor when you or your child use them.

Ultraviolet Light

Some people with eczema notice an improvement when their skin soaks up the sun. Sunlight contains ultraviolet light, which comes in three forms: UVC, which is largely absorbed by the atmosphere; UVB, which causes sunburns; and UVA, which goes through window glass and is the least harmful to the skin. There are no large, well-controlled trials of UV light on eczema, but the trials that are available show the following:

- Narrow-band UVB is superior to Broadband UVA. Narrow-band UVB is generated by a special lamp called a TL101 lamp. UVB lamps can be used at home. Ask your doctor where to buy one.
- A high dose of UVA is effective in treating eczema flares and works better than topical steroids.
- A high dose of UVA is better than UVB and UVA together. There are several ways to expose yourself to UVA rays: They are strongest below sea level in places like Death Valley, California, or the Dead Sea between Israel and Jordan. UVA rays are also generated by special lamps; ask your doctor where to find one.

PROMISING TREATMENTS

Antihistamines

Atihistamines reduce itching; however, it's still not clear why. Some researchers think it's because they sedate areas in the brain that register itch. The sedative quality of oral antihistamines can help you sleep better if taken before going to bed. Creams are also available and are preferable if you need to stay awake. Research results on antihistamines have been somewhat conflicting. What we do know is that they help some people and so far the only side effect discovered is drowsiness.

Chinese Medicine

Studies on Chinese herbal medicine have shown great benefits for adults, but not for children. These herbs are prepared individually for each patient by herbalists in areas with a large Chinese population. Herb tea is either drunk or applied to the skin. The primary problem is quality control. A good herbalist uses pure ingredients and is careful to avoid contaminants. The herbs used are Ledebouriella seseloides, Potentilla chinensis, Clematis armandii, Rehmannia glutinosa, Paeonia lactiflora, Lophatherum gracile, Dictamnus dasycarpus, Tribulus terrestris, Glycyrrhiza glabra, Schizonepeta tenuifolia, and Aneba clematidis.

Coal Tar

Coal tar is a crude mixture of hundreds of hydrocarbons. Because the mixture is so complex, the active ingredients have yet to be identified. Products made with coal tar have some drawbacks, including smell, color, and the ability to stain (black) anything it touches. Even though tar is a good and safe product, very few studies support its efficacy. Some of the newer tar preparations are much easier to apply and much less messy than the older ones.

Tar preparations come with a warning about cancer. While topical tar solutions have never been shown to cause cancer, there's a theoretical link to cancer because people in certain occupations who are exposed to tar and tar products have a higher risk of cancer.

Dietary Supplements

While eczema is not affected by the food you eat, I suspect supplements may have some influence, even though there isn't any proof that they do. Researchers think that essential fatty acids may play a role in eczema. These naturally occurring acids are involved in the production of the skin's anti-inflammatory compounds and are a primary component of the barrier. No studies proved that supplements helped eczema, but I still prescribe evening primrose oil for selected patients. Other oils like borage or fish oils may also help. Vitamins E and B_2 have been tested, and the two together appear to improve dry skin. No other supplements have shown any benefit; however, research is ongoing.

Dust Mite Desensitization

If dust mite feces are the problem, it would stand to reason that desensitizing patients with eczema would help reduce eczema. As logical as this sounds, so far research doesn't prove it one way or the other.

Dust Mite Elimination

There is strong circumstantial evidence that dust mite feces make eczema worse. I've found that eczema improves when patients live in a low dust mite environment. Eczema worsens when dust mite extracts are applied directly to the skin. Research results are mixed; however, I believe that dust mite reduction helps children more than it does adults.

Emollients

Emollients are the mainstay of eczema therapy because they replace missing oils and seal skin from external irritants. In spite of their importance in treating eczema, virtually no scientific evidence explains or supports their use.

Massage Therapy

Massage therapy is excellent for soothing and relaxing stressed eczema sufferers, regardless of age. The most effective massage comes from a trained loved one. Both parents and children are more relaxed after a massage, and it helps strengthen emotional bonds. Once again, definitive research hasn't been performed so that we can fully understand the science behind it. The beneficial effects are obvious to the participants.

TREATMENTS THAT REQUIRE MORE RESEARCH

Antimicrobial Medication

Patients with eczema are more likely to have colonies of the bacteria *Staphylococcus aureus* on their skin than those without eczema. Skin infections are common. Oral antibiotics should be used only with a severe infection, for two reasons. First, research doesn't show any benefit if there isn't an infection. Second, taking too much can build resistance. A good way to reduce skin bacteria, prevent resistance, and reduce eczema flares is to use topical antibiotics such as the prescription drug mupirocin. Topical steroids are very effective in reducing skin bacteria. Other treatments used for infections that don't seem to be effective are topical antiseptics and antifungal creams or shampoos.

Capsaicin

Capsaicin is the ingredient that causes the burn in hot foods like chili peppers. When this novel treatment is applied to long-term severe eczema, it burns at first, just as your mouth does when you eat hot food. However, capsaicin reduces Substance P, the itch chemical, and soon both burning and itching disappear.

Dust Mite Allergen Injections

Allergens are injected so that antibodies to them will be created by blood cells. This process does work for some allergies, but dust mite allergens don't seem to work for eczema.

Hospitalization

Severe, full-body eczema is a life-threatening disorder and requires hospitalization. Those with less severe eczema can benefit from a hospital stay by being removed from a stressful or flare-trigger environment.

Hypnotherapy and Biofeedback

These therapies help develop mental tools to control both the sensation of itch and the compulsion to scratch. Research on children shows that both types work quite well, especially with girls.

Interferon Gamma Injections

Interferon gamma injections are used to balance the immune system, which is characteristically skewed by eczema. In a normal immune system, the chemicals Th1 and Th2 are balanced. In those with eczema, Th2 is too strong, Th1 too weak. Following the injection of a chemical that boosts Th1, the immune system becomes balanced. This appears to help eczema; however, treatment is expensive, painful, and subject to unpleasant side effects.

Nurse Education

One study compared the benefit of a single eczema care educational session with a nurse to a visit to a dermatologist. The group that saw the nurse did better, most likely because prescribed treatments were followed more accurately and the nurses help reduce steroid use anxiety.

Platelet-Activating Factor (PAF) Antagonist

PAF is a chemical that intensifies itch when released into the skin. A treatment that inhibited or prevented its release would seem to be a good idea. The research so far doesn't show benefits from this treatment, but scientists are still working on it.

Ranitidine

Ranitidine, sold as Zantac for indigestion, is an antihistamine that also modifies immune function. Doctors using ranitidine to treat patients with ulcers who also had eczema noticed an improvement in their skin condition. Early research using ranitidine as a treatment for eczema seems to show positive results. More research is needed.

Salt Baths

Salt baths have been used for so many millennia, it's not possible to trace the origin of this treatment. We know a trip to the Dead Sea helps clear up eczema, but we don't know why. We think it's a combination of salt water and ultraviolet rays. Taking a salt bath at home so far shows the same benefit. Another study compared children with severe eczema who were taken to a beach and those who were taken to a beach with dolphins. Water with dolphins was more effective than a beach without them. So far, the reasons for this are speculative.

Suplatast Tosilate

Suplatast tosilate is currently used for asthma treatment. However, it addresses the same types of chemical processes that trigger eczema flares: the production of IgE and cytokines. Taken orally, it was shown to control the return of symptoms after steroid use had been stopped.

Oolong Tea

Drinking a liter of oolong tea consumed daily in three equal servings with meals was effective in helping patients with recalcitrant eczema. The first positive results were seen after one month, and it was still working at six months. No other type of tea was tested.

Thymic Extracts

Thymic extracts are either taken from the thymus of calves or produced synthetically as thymopentin. The idea behind its use is that people with eczema have too few T cells (T cells are produced in the thymus) and too much IgE in their blood. Researchers felt that eczema patients may benefit from a boost of thymic growth factors, which increase T cell production. While the studies have been small and badly designed, they do indicate that this would be a positive area of study. However, no research on thymic extracts has been conducted for at least ten years.

Topical Immunomodulators

TIMs are made from an interesting compound that is isolated from a bacterium. The two available today are tacrolimus

(Protopic) and pimecrolimus (Elidel). They work by deactivating T cells, which blocks the release of cytokines, the chemical that triggers itch. Tacrolimus was originally used in oral form as an immunosuppressive drug to prevent kidney and liver transplant rejection. Tacrolimus works by inhibiting T cells from talking to other cells. T cells control the immune response, so when they're blocked, the exaggerated immune response in eczema, or flares, is blocked. Tacrolimus is applied directly to the skin. Preliminary research shows this to be an exciting new treatment with few negative side effects. The only problem is that the cream tends to burn when first applied. If the medication is kept cold, this unpleasant effect is eliminated.

Concerns about an increase of skin cancer caused by using TIMs are unfounded. The incidence of cancer among those who used TIMs was actually less than expected. Doctors still recommend staying out of the sun for anyone using TIMs.

Transfer Factor

This is a white blood cell extract that boosts immunity. If eczema were an allergy, boosting immunity would make eczema worse. But many aspects of eczema suggest it's a deficiency in key components of the immune system. The one study that looked at the effects of transfer factor injections showed no significant results.

TREATMENTS WITH NO SUPPORTING RESEARCH

Aromatherapy

In an aromatherapy study, children were treated either with counseling and massage with essential oils or with counseling and massage without essential oils. Both groups improved in scores of daytime irritability and nighttime disturbance. There was no difference between the groups, which suggests the benefit of counseling and any type of massage but no benefit from aromatherapy.

Avoidance of Enzyme-Rich Detergents

Enzymes added to detergents improve cleaning power but can irritate the skin. Doctors have long suspected that such enzymes irritate eczema skin and have advised patients to avoid these products. However, the few studies that have been conducted don't support this idea. The logical conclusion is that if the detergent doesn't bother your skin, go ahead and use it regardless of enzyme content.

Bioresonance Therapy

Very popular in Europe, this treatment tries to alter the electrical and magnetic field that is produced by all people. Practitioners of bioresonance use an electronic instrument to detect perturbations in these bioelectric magnetic fields and attempt to correct the problem by reversing the pathological fields electronically. There has been one well-designed study of bioresonance that showed no effect whatsoever. This means there are no positive or negative effects.

Elimination Diets

There is a persistent myth that eczema is a food allergy. The issue has been studied exhaustively for years. While some of the studies have flawed methodology, no well-controlled scientific evidence supporting diet as a cause of eczema has ever been found.

Fabrics

There are three good trials that examine the effect of clothing on eczema. In one, cotton was reported to be the most comfortable fabric. In another, no difference was found between cotton and polyester, but all garments were uncomfortable after sweating.

Levamisole

This drug is used by veterinarians to treat worm infections. It works by stimulating the immune system to fight infection. Because patients with eczema have some problems with diminished immunity to infection and increased susceptibility to certain infections, levamisole was tested in eczema. An excellently designed study found no benefit for eczema.

Nitrazepan

Nitrazepan is widely used for sedation and as a sleeping aid. Since itching and scratching keep people awake, the idea was to help people achieve a deeper, full night's sleep with less scratching. The results of a study showed no effect on scratching, since scratching can happen while you sleep.

SUMMARY

Armed with this information, you will be able to work more effectively with your doctor. You have the right to request information about the quality or existence of research that establishes the effectiveness of the treatments or medications your doctor prescribes. Sometimes, however, what you'll hear is: "It's worked for most of my patients, even though there's been no research to show why."

Chapter Fourteen

FUTURE THERAPIES

As recently as thirty years ago, eczema affected about 10 percent of the population of northern, Westernized countries. Today, the proportion has risen to almost 20 percent, and it's still growing. For years, it was thought that eczema was the physical manifestation of emotional problems. Sufferers were prescribed psychiatric help for the underlying emotional problems, but there was little treatment or concern about the itchy rash. It would go away when the person shaped up.

This attitude has changed dramatically since the Human Genome Project revealed eczema's underlying genetic cause. Along with greater understanding of genetics and concern about eczema's growing incidence is a heightened interest in further research. More and more scientists are studying this uncomfortable but not fatal disorder.

Therapies for eczema are being sought in academic laboratories, the research and development facilities of personal care product companies, and pharmaceutical companies' labs. Because of the enormous financial rewards expected from finding a powerful treatment or cure for eczema, many teams keep their research secret until it's tested and patented. However, interested doctors hear rumors, and the news circulating is good.

RESEARCH IN PREVENTIVE TREATMENTS

Preventive treatments can either keep eczema from developing in the first place, stop eczema from progressing to severe eczema, or prevent the onset of asthma or rhinitis.

Research on Infant and Maternal Diet

Since popular opinion asserts that eczema is caused by an allergic food reaction, researchers are studying expectant mothers who already have a child with eczema. The research looks at these questions:

- Does avoidance of certain foods prevent eczema?
- Does exposing infants to certain foods at an early age make them tolerant?
- Does dietary intervention delay the onset of eczema or decrease its severity?
- Do the advantages of food intervention outweigh the complexities of managing a specific diet?
- Does exclusive breast-feeding prevent eczema?
- Does prolonged breast-feeding prevent eczema?
- Does the early introduction of solid foods cause eczema?
- What impact does the mother's diet have on a nursing baby?

While these questions might seem simple, finding good answers in double-blind studies is not. Along with the difficulty of finding mothers and babies to participate is the problem of ending up with skewed results, since not all mothers breastfeed.

Other research has been done on the diet of pregnant women and their exposure to allergens. So far, the few, small studies done show no significant results. The interest in this research is as much to lay to rest folk wisdom as it is to find influences on the development of eczema.

Probiotics

Probiotic therapy, where babies are fed good germs, is based on the idea that many infants are kept in an overly clean environment. Lack of exposure to germs and pollen prevents the child's immune system from developing properly. This promising research has shown results; however, more research is needed.

Early Treatment

Research is being conducted to see if early treatment of eczema prevents the onset of asthma and rhinitis. Preliminary results suggest this may be true. If continuing research holds, it means that managing eczema, a non-life-threatening disorder, will either prevent the development or reduce the severity of asthma, which is a potentially life-threatening disease.

Vaccines

Vaccines have been used to prevent polio, measles, and a host of other diseases. Promising research from New Zealand suggests that one type of vaccine may be useful in treating children with severe atopic dermatitis. Since the research is proprietary, details aren't available, but a first look at early results is encouraging.

Itch Research

In addition to research on eczema itself, some scientists have focused on the mechanism of itch. Itching isn't fatal, so research dollars aren't pouring into labs that explore this interesting topic. However, for some scientists it's a fascinating subject, and research is being done. One promising area is research into the chemicals that carry messages from one cell to another. It's possible that itching is triggered by miscommunication among cells. Too many messages may be sent or sent to the wrong place. Or perhaps the message is received correctly but then passed on in the wrong direction. Research on cell communication is in the very early stages, and so far scientists have been unable to pinpoint the chemicals sending itch signals. The next generation of itch treatments will be potent, selective, and long-lasting. If we can cure the itch, we will go a long way toward curing the misery, and rash, of eczema. To learn more about itch research, go to www.itchforum.org.

ATTACKING THE SYMPTOMS

Artificial Barriers

Artificial barriers are lotions applied to the skin that fill in the breaks in the stratum corneum. These products originated primarily to protect workers' hands from dangerous chemicals without forcing them to wear bulky gloves. The product is a gift to those with hand eczema. A product such as Gloves in a Bottle is absorbed into the outer layer of skin and bonds to it. It doesn't wash off; it is sloughed off just like normal skin.

Aids for Faulty Barriers

Scientists in personal care products companies are trying to develop better moisturizers. Procter & Gamble has developed a product that cleans and moisturizes the skin. The moisturizer doesn't rub off when toweling.

In the future, moisturizers will be smarter. They'll balance the body's own natural lipid content and restore the barrier, matching deficiency with the amount of moisturizer necessary. In the beginning, there may be only a few barrier creams that would be used for most skin types. As technology progresses, it may be possible to have a moisturizer formulated specifically for you.

Oral Solutions

Protecting a faulty barrier with a pill is still a dream. While research is ongoing, no one has found a pill that doesn't have unwanted side effects. At the moment, doctors prescribe evening primrose oil, vitamin B_3, and vitamin C for both eczema and essential fatty acid deficiency. It may not be possible to fit all the oil your body needs into a single pill; however, coming up with a medicine that would stimulate the skin to produce the missing elements is possible.

TIMs

Topical immunomodulators are showing great promise in treating eczema by inhibiting the production of cytokine, the itch chemical. Newer oral immunomodulators are being developed that are more powerful but have fewer side effects.

Biologics

Biologic medications, or *biologics,* are developed from living sources, such as cells, rather than the chemicals of current drugs. These targeted medications are designed to block or eliminate immune cells that cause outbreaks of eczema. Biologics are relatively new, and their long-term safety isn't known. Still, they are an important new treatment option, and they may be available soon for eczema. An existing biologic therapy for asthma is now being tested for use in eczema. The brand name is Xolair, made by Novartis.

Defensins

Defensins are naturally occurring proteins in the skin that protect against infection. They are used in the opposite way from biologics. These drugs support, rather than suppress, immune response. By attacking bacteria, defensin medication supports the destruction of staph and other bacteria.

Inhibiting Toll Receptors

Toll receptors trigger other cells to release cytokines, which in turn trigger itching. The simple act of washing your hands can set off the toll receptors. Research into soaps and cleansers that prevent the activation of toll receptors is ongoing. So far, there aren't any products on the market, but there may be some soon.

Peptides

Researchers have recently identified a number of small, biologically active peptides that promote healing in the skin. Research is ongoing to find a way to use these peptides to build up the barrier layer.

Acidic Hot Salty Water (Balneotherapy)

It has been known for centuries that acidic, hot, salty baths are a miracle cure for eczema. The Dead Sea was used as a therapeutic spot by the ancient Greeks. Even though a dip in water like the Dead Sea has been known to provide a dramatic reduction in eczema, little research has been done to find out why. Researchers are currently looking into this interesting phenomenon.

CURE

The goal of a cure is to get rid of eczema permanently. The tool for finding this holy grail is understanding the genetic causes of eczema. Currently, parents can be tested to see if their child is at risk. In the future, scientists will be able to distinguish among types of eczema and then create a targeted cure for each type.

Gene Therapy

Gene therapy is in its infancy, but it's making progress at an enormous rate. Eczema results when myriad genes don't function properly. Since so many genes are involved, creating a cure targeted at eczema only is still in the future.

• • •

Breakthroughs in science can happen at any time. New treatments for eczema are frequently released for public use. As an interested party, it's a good idea to keep tabs on these developments. You never know; the cure that will permit you to live eczema-free could be just around the corner.

Glossary

Abscess: A collection of pus under the skin, usually associated with bacterial infection. Can appear as a red, raised bump under the skin. It is often warm and tender. It is typically walled off from the outside world but can occasionally drain foul-smelling yellow or green thick fluid.

Acne: Inflammation of the pilosebaceous units of the skin (hair follicles and their associated oil glands), leading to white-heads, blackheads, pimples, nodules, cysts. Cysts and nodules can be painful. Acne is often scarring and disfiguring.

Allergen: A foreign substance that causes an allergic reaction (for example, pollen is an allergen).

Allergic Contact Dermatitis: A rash of the skin caused by an allergic reaction to an externally applied substance. For example, nickel dermatitis is a contact allergy to nickel, which is found in alloyed jewelry.

Allergy: A reaction by the immune system to a foreign substance that is inappropriate and out of proportion to the concentration of the foreign substance. For example, a peanut allergy can cause widespread symptoms to minute quantities of peanut allergens. Allergies are also highly specific. For example, someone allergic to peanuts will not necessarily react to all nuts, or someone allergic to dog hair may not be allergic to cat hair.

Antibody: Defense protein made by the immune system's B cells. It binds and neutralizes foreign substances. Comes in five types: IgA, IgE, IgM, IgG, and IgD.

Asteatotic Eczema: An eczemalike reaction seen on the lower legs, particularly of the elderly, due to extremely dry skin and poor circulation.

Atopic: Literally meaning "no place." Refers to a tendency to develop immune hypersensitivity, particularly in the skin, the lungs, and the nasal passages (*see* Atopic Triad). Atopy is typically hereditary.

Atopic Dermatitis: A hereditary, intensely itchy, inflammatory condition of the skin. It can be acute, subacute, or chronic (lifelong). It is associated with inflammation of the epidermis and dermis. There may or may not be an associated family history of asthma, rhinitis, hay fever, and atopic dermatitis. Atopic dermatitis differs based upon the person's age. Different rash distributions and types are seen in infancy, childhood, and adults, although there is considerable overlap.

Atopic Triad: The tendency of atopic diseases to cluster together in individuals or families.

Atopy: The tendency to develop atopic conditions.

Atrophy: Thinning of the skin, a common side effect of prolonged use of potent steroids, particularly in sensitive areas.

B Cell: A cell of the immune system, made in the bone marrow, responsible for producing antibodies.

Balneotherapy: A form of treatment where mineral baths are taken with or without additional treatment (such as sun exposure). An example includes treatments at resorts along the Dead Sea, where the high mineral concentration of the sea water is combined with the special form of sunlight that penetrates the surrounding shore (high in UVA because the Dead Sea is below sea level) to treat psoriasis. This type of treatment is beneficial for eczema as well.

Barrier: The outermost portion of the epidermis, which is responsible for keeping harmful substances out of and moisture in the skin. The barrier is composed of lipid, protein, and tightly interwoven layers of mummified cells of the extreme external epidermis. When the barrier is damaged (either from atopic dermatitis, from exposure to irritants, or both), irritants and allergens can penetrate the epidermis and dermis, where they trigger immune responses leading to itch, scratch, and allergy.

Basophil: A cell of the immune system, made in the bone marrow, responsible for making histamine, the key component of itch.

Bathing: A process of hydrating the epidermis. In eczema, the purpose of bathing is not to cleanse the skin, it is to add moisture back. Therefore, bathing may be performed in warm water and should be done for at least 15 minutes. To seal in the moisture, emollients need to be applied within 3 minutes of exiting the bath; otherwise, evaporation depletes the epidermis of too much moisture and defeats the process.

Biopsy of Skin: A minor surgical procedure designed to diagnose skin disease. The procedure is done under local anesthesia. Anesthetic is injected into the skin either directly (slightly painful) or after the skin has been prenumbed with a special anesthetic cream (less painful). Once the skin is numb, either a scalpel blade or a special punch tool (which resembles a round cookie cutter) is used to obtain the specimen. Specimen size varies but for eczema is typically 6 millimeters or less (25 millimeters to 1 inch). The risks of skin biopsies include pain, infection, and scarring (which may be permanent) but tend to be low.

Blepharitis: Redness, scaling, and itching of the eyelids. This is common in eczema or allergic contact dermatitis of the face.

Bone Marrow: The spongy living material in the cores of the long bones of the body. The bone marrow is a factory that makes blood and all components of the immune system, including B cells, T cells, Langerhans cells, mast cells, basophils, and eosinophils. The bone marrow also makes red blood cells, which transport oxygen, and platelets, which aid in clotting.

Bulla: A large blister, commonly seen in severe allergic contact dermatitis, severe eczema, particularly on the lower legs, or certain infections, such as bullous impetigo. **Bullae** can develop from toxic exposures to the skin (severe sunburn, chemical burn, and physical burn, and severe dermatitis from poison ivy).

Candida: A yeast. In eczema, yeast infections can occur anywhere on the skin, not just the vaginal area. They tend to favor areas that are warm and moist, such as the armpits and groin, as well as skin folds below the breasts and the abdominal fat rolls. They can also occur between the fingers and toes. Candida infections are red, itchy, and scaly. The skin is often whitish, mushy, and waterlogged (a condition called *maceration*).

Cellulitis: Typically, a bacterial infection of the deeper tissues of the skin. The skin appears red, is not tender, and is sometimes firm. People can often have a fever with cellulitis. On the limbs, cellulitis often tracks up toward the body in red streaks. This is a serious sign requiring intravenous antibiotics.

Cold Sore: Also known as a fever blister. This is typically a collection of tiny blisters, usually around the mouth, that are caused by herpes simplex virus infection. Cold sores are painful and tend to recur in the same location. Occasionally, they can be accompanied by malaise, fever, and swollen glands (lymph nodes) near the location of the blister. Cold sores can be triggered by stress, sunlight, immune suppression, and certain medications. In eczema, cold sores are taken seriously because they are associated with eczema herpeticum, a condition where herpes simplex virus spreads like wildfire over the whole body. People with eczema herpeticum can require hospitalization.

Contact Dermatitis: A dermatitislike rash caused by external agents.

Allergic: The external agent is an allergen.
Irritant: The external agent is an irritant.
Hand: Contact dermatitis localized to the hands.
Occupational: Contact dermatitis due to work-related exposure.

Corticosteroid: A naturally occurring hormone responsible for a number of normal body functions. There are several different natural or endogenous corticosteroids that regulate everything from growth (anabolic steroids), to sexual differentiation and function (testosterone and estrogen), to salt balance and blood pressure maintenance (mineralocorticoids), to the "fight or flight" response to stress. Synthetic corticosteroids are chemically modified versions that are used by drugmakers to target specific functions. Corticosteroids used in eczema suppress the immune system. They inhibit the activity of B cells and T cells. They are associated with side effects. However, if used properly and on a short-term basis, they are a valuable tool in quenching eczema flares. Repeated used of oral corticosteroids is not recommended for eczema because 1) the risk of side effects is too high; 2) the eczema becomes "brittle" or unresponsive to ever higher doses of oral corticosteroids; and 3) eczema tends to relapse more quickly and to a greater degree.

Cradle Cap: A condition in infants associated with yellow, greasy, and occasionally itchy scale of the scalp.

Cytokine: A small molecule used by cells of the immune system to talk to one another. Some cytokines also talk with nerves, the spinal cord, and the brain, thus integrating the immune system and the nervous system. They are an important component of itch and the itch-scratch cycle.

Dermatitis: A red, angry, inflamed rash.

Asteatotic: Localized to the lower legs, particularly in older men.

Atopic: Location depends on age, severity depends on chronicity.

Contact: Due to external exposure.

Dyshidrotic: Made up largely of vesicles, normally hands and feet.

Seborrheic: Associated with a yellow, greasy scale and less itch.

Dermatophytosis: Infection of the skin with dermatophyte fungus.

Dermis: The middle layer of skin; contains collagen, blood vessels, lymphatics, nerves, and spongy tissue bathed in fluid. Interspersed in the fluid are cells such as fibroblasts (which make collagen) and very few mast cells. Cells of the immune system (T cells, B cells, Langerhans cells, eosinophils, and basophils) can traffic here in massive numbers during an inflammatory response. They can bring a lot of fluid with them to cause swelling of the tissue as well.

Eczema: A red, angry, inflamed rash.

Atopic: Location depends on age, severity depends on chronicity.

Asteatotic: Localized to the lower legs, particularly in older men.

Contact: Due to external exposure.

Craquelatum: With a predominantly dried mud flat appearance.

Discoid: Synonym for nummular; means round or disk shaped.

Dyshidrotic: Made up largely of vesicles, normally on hands and feet.

Nummular: Synonym for dyshidrotic; means coin shaped.

Emollient: A topically applied substance containing some combination of oil mixed with water. Its purpose is to lubricate skin, to soothe irritated skin, to trap moisture in a well-hydrated epidermis, and to serve as a substitute for the lipid component of the barrier until the skin's own barrier can be repaired naturally. Bland (lacking preservatives, additives, or fragrances) emollients are an essential component of daily eczema therapy.

Eosinophil: A cell of the immune system that contains granules of powerful proteins inside it. The proteins are released when IgE bound to allergen comes into contact with the eosinophil. Normally, eosinophils fight parasitic infections. In diseases, they can mount inappropriate allergic responses, which lead to conditions like asthma, allergic rhinitis, and food allergy. Although eosinophils may be elevated in patients with atopic dermatitis, they do not appear to be associated with any allergy. However, patients with atopic dermatitis are vulnerable to developing other allergic diseases as part of the atopic triad (such as rhinitis and asthma). Food allergy is extremely rare in eczema.

Epidermis: The outer layer of the skin. It contains nerve endings, melanocytes (pigment-producing cells), Langerhans cells, keratinocytes, and the barrier. Under the right conditions (an eczema flare), the epidermis can team with cells of the immune system such as T cells, B cells, and Langerhans cells.

Erythema: Redness visible on the skin due to blood vessel dilation and increased blood flow in the dermis; one of the hallmarks of inflammation.

Erythroderma: Widespread erythema of the skin, often with no area of the body spared.

Fever Blister: *See* Cold Sore.

Fissure: A crack in the skin. Microscopic fissures cannot be seen, but their existence has been inferred by studies that measure impairment of barrier function. Superficial fissures go into the epidermis, medium fissures to the dermis (drawing blood). Deep fissures extend to the subcutis and are unlikely to heal without medical attention. Fissures pose a risk for itch and infection.

Flat Wart: A skin infection caused by human papillomavirus, resulting in flat, skin-colored, slightly rough bumps on the skin. They range in size from 1 to 6 millimeters or larger. Flat warts can occur in isolation, they can be scattered, or they can occur in clustered groups anywhere on the skin. They can number from one to hundreds.

Folliculitis: Infection of hair follicles.

Bacterial: Caused by bacteria.

Candidal: Caused by the yeast candida.

Dermatophytic: Caused by dermatophyte fungus.

Staphylococcal: Caused by the bacteria staph.

Fungal Infection: An infection caused by a fungus, yeast, or mold.

Candidiasis: Caused by yeast.

Dermatophytosis: Caused by fungus.

Onychomycosis: Fungal infection of the nails.

Pityriasis versicolor: A fungus caused by the organism Malassezia furfur.

Hand Eczema: Eczema localized to the hands. It typically occurs in people at risk for eczema who wash their hands frequently: health care workers, young mothers, mechanics.

Herpes Simplex Virus: The principal virus responsible for cold sores.

Histamine: A small molecule that induces itch; it also stimulates blood vessels to dilate. The latter can contribute to redness and swelling.

Human Papillomavirus: The virus responsible for warts.

Humectant: A substance that can hold water like a sponge. While emollients seal in the water already in the epidermis, humectants suck water out of their surroundings. Putting a humectant on the skin pulls water out of the air (external environment) and out of the dermis (internal environment) to hydrate the epidermis. Examples of humectants are lactic acid, glycolic acid, and urea. Good humectants also loosen tightly adherent keratinocytes and promote exfoliation. They are a good way to get rid of scale.

Ichthyosis: A scaly condition caused by inappropriate accumulation of keratinocytes that adhere too tightly and do not slough off normally. The result is scale and an impaired barrier. Ichthyosis vulgaris is very common in eczema.

IgE (Immunoglobulin E): One of five types of antibodies made by B cells. It is particularly relevant for allergic reactions to pollen, mold, and foods.

Immune System: A complex defense network of the body. It coordinates the actions of organs (the bone marrow, the lymph nodes, the spleen, the thymus), cells (B cells, T cells, Langerhans cells), proteins (antibodies), and small molecules (cytokines) to defend the body against any and all forms of attack. When the immune system breaks down, we are vulnerable to attack. When the immune system turns against the body, we develop autoimmune disease (like lupus or rheumatoid arthritis). When the immune system is overactive against foreign substances, we develop hypersensitivity or allergy.

Immunoglobulin: A protein that recognizes a foreign substance. The body, through its B cells, makes a library of millions and millions of different immunoglobulins, each of which falls into one of five classes (*see* Antibody). Each particular B cell makes only one particular type of immunoglobulin—for example, one recognizing peanut allergen. The B cell can switch the immunoglobulin to any class of its choosing (for example, IgA to peanut allergen, or IgD to peanut allergen, or IgE to peanut allergen, and so forth). Each different class operates in a different context. For atopy, IgE is the most important.

Impetigo: A specific bacterial infection of the skin caused by staph accumulating in the epidermis. The skin is red and covered with a yellow honey crust. Impetigo can also have blisters and bullae.

Inflammation: In the skin, an immune reaction leading to redness, swelling, pain, itch, possible fever, and possible loss of function (for instance, if the digits are involved and can't bend from too much swelling).

Irritant: A corrosive substance that damages the skin and can cause a rash. While allergens can operate at very low concentrations, irritants are concentration-dependent. High concentrations of irritants cause more severe rashes than low concentrations of irritants. Examples of irritants include sulfuric acid and harsh soaps. Irritants can break down the skin's barrier and make it more vulnerable to allergens.

Itch: An uncomfortable sensation that leads to the desire to scratch.

Keloid: A thick, raised scar, often located on certain areas of the body in people predisposed to developing keloids (particularly Hispanics and African Americans). Areas prone to developing keloids are the ears, the central chest, the shoulders, and the back.

Keratinocyte: The principal cell of the epidermis.

Langerhans Cell: A cell of the immune system that traffics from the blood to the skin to the lymph nodes and back. Langerhans cells have many tentacles that trap foreign substances. They then process these substances so that they can be presented to cells of the immune system in the lymph nodes. Once they "show" the foreign invader to T cells or B cells, the induce a vigorous and specific immune response to that substance.

Lichen Simplex Chronicus: A chronic form of eczema associated with lichenification.

Lichenification: Thickening of the skin from repeated rubbing or scratching.

Lipid: An oil-soluble substance. An important component of the barrier. Examples include ceramide and cholesterol. Artificial barrier creams attempt to reproduce the skin's natural lipid content. To date, there is no cream that perfectly mimics the skin's own barrier lipids.

Lymph: A clear fluid that contains interstitial fluid (the water between cells and tissues), cells of the immune system, and any foreign substances that have entered the body. Lymph circulates in a parallel circulatory system just like the blood's circulatory system. It starts in tissues, goes via lymphatic channels, is filtered through a series of lymph nodes, and drains into the bloodstream. Blood then goes out to the tissues. In the tiniest blood vessels, the capillaries, tiny bits of clear fluid squeeze out through microscopic holes in the capillaries and wash through the tissues, where the cycle starts all over again. Lymph is essentially an ultrafiltrate of blood and immune cells.

Lymph Node: Also known as *glands,* these are tiny rubbery balls of tissue (1 to 10 millimeters) containing T cells, B cells, and Langerhans cells. They are constantly bathed in lymph, a fluid that washes through every tissue in the body and drains into lymph nodes via lymphatic channels. Lymph nodes filter lymph for foreign substances. If any are trapped, they are presented to the immune system for review. If they are recognized as being harmful, an immune response is mounted against them. If they are recognized as innocuous, they are allowed to pass through these chains of filters to the bloodstream.

Lymphatic Channel: A thin-walled vessel analogous to the blood vessel, except it carries lymph.

Lymphocyte: A cell commonly found in lymph, ordinarily either a T cell or a B cell.

Macule: A flat, small area of rash on the skin.

Mast Cell: A histamine-producing cell made in the bone marrow and found in the dermis.

Melanin: Pigment made by melanocytes.

Melanocyte: Pigment-producing cells that give skin its color.

Mold: A type of fungus.

Molluscum Contagiosum: A viral infection caused by a poxvirus that makes red pinpoint bumps on the skin. It can easily be spread from one part of the body to another and is more difficult to spread from one person to another. This type of infection is more commonly seen in eczema.

Mycosis Fungoides: A skin cancer of T cells flooding the dermis and epidermis. It can sometimes mimic eczema.

Nerve: A threadlike extension of a nerve cell (neuron) that ends in a receptor. The receptor may be for pain, itch, vibration, pressure, heat, cold, or another nerve cell (for example, in the spinal cord or brain). Nerves can be stimulated by chemicals, cytokines, and physical stimuli (such as pressure, being cut, or scratched).

Nickel Dermatitis: An allergic contact dermatitis caused by nickel.

Nipple Eczema: A type of eczema common on the nipples and areolae of men and women, particularly joggers with eczema. Nipple eczema that doesn't heal in 3 weeks of treatment should be tested for Paget's disease, a rare form of breast cancer.

Nodule: A bump under the skin. It is often easier to feel than to see.

Nummular Eczema: Coin-shaped eczema, often found in the lower extremities in adults and more common in men. It can be found anywhere in children, both boys and girls.

Onychomycosis: Fungal infection of the nails.

Papillomavirus: *See* Human Papillomavirus.

Papule: A small raised bump on the skin (less than 1 centimeter).

Parasitosis: Infestation of the skin with a bug.

Patch Testing: A technique used to determine contact allergy. Patches containing various allergens are applied to the skin. Within 48 hours, the patches are removed, and results are read anywhere from immediately to 96 hours later. Allergic contact dermatitis is less common in eczema, although nickel dermatitis is frequently seen.

Pediculus humanus capitis: Head lice. They can cause itchy scalp and minimal rash.

Pediculus humanus corporis: Body lice. They can cause widespread itching and little rash.

Phthirus pubis: Pubic lice. They can cause itching in the pubic area.

Perioral Dermatitis: Acnelike rash occurring around the mouth, nose, and sometimes the eyes. It can also be red, slightly flaky, and itchy. One cause is inappropriate use of steroids or very thick, pore-clogging moisturizers on the face. It can be difficult to treat and may occasionally require prolonged therapy with oral antibiotics.

Phototherapy: Treatment using ultraviolet light. Patients are exposed to ultraviolet lights that look like fluorescent lights, except they emit a bluish hue. Light units can be small to treat just the hands or feet. There are wall units that can treat one-half of the body at a time, and there are enclosures that treat the body from all sides simultaneously (the latter may be impractical for people who are claustrophobic). Lights are labeled based upon the wavelength (portion of the light spectrum) emitted by the bulbs. Ultraviolet light comes in three principal wavelengths: UVA, UVB, and UVC. UVA is ineffective at treating eczema and it must be combined with a light-activated medication such as Psoralen to be effective; hence the name PUVA (Psoralen UVA) therapy. The combination does increase the risk of skin cancer and cataracts (opacities of the lenses of the eyes). UVB is effective for treating eczema. Narrow-band UVB, a subset of UVB light, can be dissected out. This is the most selective for treating eczema and has the fewest side effects. Narrow-band UVB is gaining greater acceptance as a potent yet relatively safe treatment for severe eczema. UVC is not used therapeutically.

Pityriasis Alba: A whitish discoloration of the skin found in people of color who have eczema. Typical locations include the face and arms, although any body surface area can be involved. Pityriasis alba is reversible; if the eczema is treated, the color returns to normal.

Pityriasis Versicolor: A fungal infection causing skin color changes: red, white, pink, and brown. It is more common in hot and humid environments and during the summer. Skin color changes resolve once the fungus is treated. Diagnosis is made by scraping off flakes of skin and analyzing them under the microscope. It can occasionally be confused with pityriasis alba, but pityriasis alba shows no fungal organisms under the microscope.

Plaque: A large portion of skin (greater than 1 centimeter).

Poison Ivy Dermatitis: An allergic reaction caused by exposure to poison ivy. The rash is typically red and weepy, with linear streaks suggestive of brushing against a plant. It can occur 1 to 3 days following exposure to the plant. The causative agent is a plant oil called *urushiol*, which is clear or yellowish and is found in the sap of the plant. The rash can occur indirectly from contact with clothing, tools, or pets exposed to the oil. Burning the plant can lead to aerosolization of urushiol, which can cause a skin rash as well as inflammation of the airways and lungs. The latter can rarely be fatal.

Pompholyx: A type of eczema, usually of the hands and feet, characterized by intense itching and blister formation. Redness is less common. Bouts can last from 1 to 2 weeks and are followed by clear periods lasting from weeks to months.

Prick Testing: A type of allergy test where tiny quantities (0.1 cubic centimeter) of allergen are injected into the skin (intradermal prick test) or are introduced into tiny pinpricks on the surface of the skin (epicutaneous prick test) to test for an allergic response. An allergic response typically shows up as a bump or wheal at the prick or injection site. Allergens include pollens, molds, plants, foods, and pets. Positive responses are strongly suggestive of allergy. Negative responses suggest but do not prove lack of allergy. There is a remote chance of anaphylactic shock from this type of testing, so it needs to take place at a facility where emergency resuscitation can be performed if necessary.

Prurigo Nodularis: A skin condition of unknown cause, thought to be worsened by stress, characterized by itchy knots on the skin ranging from 0.51 centimeter. Knots can persist for years and are quite difficult to treat. They are almost always located on areas of the body that can be reached. Common locations include the scalp, arms, and legs. The knots scar when healed, often permanently.

Pruritus: The Latin and scientific term for itch. Note the spelling. Unlike dermatitis, pruritus ends in *-us*.

Psoriasis: A hereditary skin condition characterized by scaly red plaques, mostly on the elbows, knees, and the scalp. It may or may not be itchy and may or may not involve the joints (psoriatic arthritis). A small number of people have very itchy psoriasis and eczema coexisting. Some of the genes that cause psoriasis are shared with the genes that cause eczema.

Pustule: A transparent, dome-shaped bump on the skin filled with infected yellowish fluid. Most often the fluid contains bacteria, but it may contain fungi or viruses.

PUVA: Psoralen ultraviolet A, or PUVA, therapy is a way to treat some forms of skin disease. It entails swallowing a tablet of a medication called Psoralen, waiting a defined period for the medication to be absorbed and make its way to the skin, and then exposing the skin to ultraviolet light in the UVA portion of the spectrum. The eyes and skin need to be protected from sunlight for 24 hours after therapy. Treatments are given 2 to 3 times weekly for several weeks. It is very effective for treating severe eczema flares and can result in remissions that last for many months. Risks include eye damage (cataracts) and skin cancers with cumulative exposure. Side effects of the medication include nausea, gastrointestinal upset, vomiting, and occasionally diarrhea.

Rash: A temporary change in the skin. Rashes come in all shapes, sizes, colors, and locations. Temporary means weeks, months, and occasionally years. Each disease may have its own rash, or several different diseases may share a similar rash. Rashes are described by their appearance and then sorted into the disease they fall under. For example, chicken pox may have papules, vesicles, pustules, bullae, or crusts. The disease is chicken pox, and its rash consists of bumps, blisters, pus bumps, and scabs. Eczema has papules, patches, vesicles, scale, erythema, fissuring, lichenification, erosions, excoriations, and crust. The disease is eczema, and its rash consists of bumps, areas of skin of a separate color or texture, blisters, redness, cracking, thickening, scratches, and scabs. The rash of eczema changes depending upon age (infant vs. child vs. adult, see pages 231–232) and depending upon how long it's been going on (acute, hours/days; subacute, days/weeks; chronic, weeks/months or longer).

RAST: Radioallergosorbent test, a blood test designed to detect circulating in the bloodstream antibodies to known allergens such as foods, pollens, molds, insects, and pets. A sample of blood is drawn and analyzed for the presence of these circulating antibodies. A positive test does not necessarily mean allergy, and a negative test does not always mean lack of allergy.

Ringworm: A lay term for tinea, or dermatophyte fungus infection of the skin. So-called because lesions start as small bumps that grow into large flat scaly circles. The center of the circle clears back to normal skin, while the edges grow outward so that the lesion resembles a doughnut or a ring. These infections can occur anywhere on the body (tinea capitis occurs on the scalp; tinea corporis on the body; tinea cruris in the groin; tinea pedis on the feet; tinea manuum on the hands; tinea unguium in the nails).

Scabies: Intensely itchy rash caused by a tiny mite *(Sarcoptes scabiei)*. It is spread by close contact with someone who is infected. The rash of scabies is often minimal and frequently missed. Typical locations of the rash are the hands, the web spaces of the fingers and toes, the wrists and ankles, and the groin area. It is commonly known as the "seven-year itch." It is more common in day care and nursing home settings but can occur anywhere. Treatments for eczema suppress the immune system and may mask or worsen scabies.

Scratch: Using the nails, a blunt instrument, or a sharp instrument to repeatedly dig at a source of itching. The act may or may not break the skin. Rubbing is a sublimated form of scratching.

Seborrheic Dermatitis: A common chronic skin condition featuring redness and yellowish, greasy scale on the parts of the body where the oil-producing glands (sebaceous glands) are most active. This includes the scalp, face (eyebrows, around the nose, cheeks, and chin), and upper chest. In infants, this condition is called *cradle cap;* in adults, in the scalp, it has been called *dandruff*.

Spleen: A principal organ of the immune system. It resides on the left upper belly in most individuals and is directly connected to the blood supply. It is a filter for infectious organisms and foreign bodies circulating in the bloodstream. It also sends retired blood cells to the scrap heap for recycling.

Staphylococcal Infections: Infections caused by the bacterium *Staphylococcus aureus.*

Abscess
Carbuncle
Furuncle
Cellulitis
Folliculitis
Impetigo

Stasis Dermatitis: Red, scaly, itchy rash of the lower legs, often occurring in elderly individuals with poor leg circulation. It may occur in younger people whose leg circulation is impaired from injury or in individuals with chronic varicose veins.

Streptococcal Infections: Infections caused by the bacterium *Streptococcus pyogenes.*

Erysipelas: painful, red, hot areas of skin caused by direct entry of bacteria through a tiny break in the skin.
Impetigo: a yellow honey crust, often itchy, scabby area surrounded by redness caused by direct entry of the bacteria through a tiny break in the skin.

Subcutis: The deepest layer of skin, bounded above by the dermis and below by fascia and muscle. This layer contains mostly fat and is insulating, shock-absorbing, and a storage depot for energy.

T Cell: A type of white blood cell involved in immune defense. It is born in the bone marrow, educated in the thymus, and sent out into the bloodstream and the skin to search for and neutralize enemies. T cells are the quarterbacks of the immune system. They tell other cells (such as B cells) what to do. They communicate with one another and the rest of the immune system through cytokines. T cells come in several varieties. Normally, the varieties are balanced (for example, Th1 equals Th2). In some diseases, there is an imbalance of subsets of T cells. For example, in eczema there is a preponderance of Th2 cells. New eczema treatments are targeting the T cell either to reduce its numbers (so there aren't enough T cells to mount an eczema response) or to restore balance (either by boosting Th1 or suppressing Th2).

Thymus: An organ in the neck that is very large in infants (the size of a fist) and gradually shrinks by early adolescence (pea size). The thymus selects T cells passing through it for duty. Those fit for duty are allowed to live; those that aren't don't make it through. Being fit for duty means a number of things: learning to fight against foreign invaders, learning not to fight against the self, and being able to properly communicate with other cells in the immune system. Some observers have likened the thymus to a classroom whose purpose is to educate T cells. Those that make a passing grade get to graduate. Unlike the case for school, those that fail are doomed.

Tinea: Fungal infection of the skin.

Barbae: affecting the beard area.

Capitis: affecting the scalp and scalp hair.

Corporis: affecting the body.
Cruris: affecting the groin (jock itch).
Facialis: affecting the face.
Manuum: affecting the hands.
Pedis: affecting the feet (athlete's foot).
Unguium: affecting the nails.
Versicolor

Ulcer: A stomach ulcer is a hole in the lining of the stomach. A skin ulcer is a hole in the lining of the skin (the epidermis).

Ultraviolet Radiation: A portion of the light spectrum. When white light or sunlight is divided into its component colors, a rainbow appears. One end is red, the other is blue. Beyond the visible portion of blue and violet lies ultraviolet light. This light makes up only a small fraction of the total spectrum of light hitting the earth, but it packs the most energy when it comes to skin. Ultraviolet light can damage the skin, causing sunburn and skin cancer as well as photoaging. When harnessed properly, ultraviolet light can be used therapeutically. If administered in carefully controlled doses, it can treat even the worst forms of eczema. Even under controlled conditions, though, there are risks, and these need to be balanced with the severity of the eczema and the risks of other therapies. Ultraviolet light impairs the skin's immune system. It increases the number of immune-suppressive cytokines and reduces the numbers of immune-activating Langerhans cells. This combination is a very powerful way to suppress eczema. Because only the skin immune system is targeted, only eczema is affected, and overall immunity is unimpaired.

UVA
UVB
Narrow-band UVB

Urticaria: Commonly known as *hives*. Red wheals on the skin that can be itchy. They appear the way inflamed mosquito bites may appear. Hives are not caused by eczema and are not a classic feature of eczema. They are treated with antihistamines.

Verruca: Latin for wart.

Vesicle: A small, fluid-filled, dome-shaped transparent bump on the skin (less than 0.5 centimeter).

Viral Infection

Human papillomavirus: The virus causing warts.

Molluscum contagiosum: The virus causing molluscum lesions.

Herpes simplex virus: The virus responsible for cold sores and genital herpes.

Vitiligo: Permanent (if untreated) white discoloration of the skin from absence of melanocytes.

Warts: Skin infection caused by human papillomavirus.

Common

Condyloma acuminatum: genital warts.

Flat

Plantar: warts on the soles of the feet.

Wheal: A raised red welt on the skin, similar to that seen in urticaria.

Yeast: A single-celled infectious organism that can cause a number of conditions depending upon location: thrush in the mouth, vaginal yeast infection, rash in the groin, nail yeast infections, and infections in the skin folds. Typically yeast infections show red, itchy skin, with an overlying subtle or quite pronounced whitish, cheesy material. There can also be small, whitish pustules at the periphery of the rash. Yeast infections are common in warm, moist areas of skin like the skin folds. These areas are also prone to getting eczema. Eczema treatments can worsen yeast infections, so it's good to check for yeast in these areas if eczema is not improving.

Zinc Deficiency: A rare condition that results in a red, scaly, not terribly itchy rash around the mouth and genital area, hands, and feet. It can occasionally be mistaken for eczema or seborrheic dermatitis. Other findings include hair loss and diarrhea. It's more common in infants, especially when children are placed on cow's milk after being weaned from breast milk. Zinc supplementation completely clears the rash and other symptoms.

Resources

MEDICAL DICTIONARY/TERMINOLOGY

- The University of Iowa College of Medicine's Department of Dermatology offers a wealth of information on skin disease and eczema. The information is appropriate for both the general reader and the specialist: tray.dermatology.uiowa.edu.
- The National Institutes of Health (NIH) has information about eczema and other skin disorders as well as information on current research. Their Web site is www.nlm.nih.gov/medlineplus/skindiseasesgeneral.html.
- The University of Maryland lists eighty common dermatologic terms and definitions at www.umm.edu/dermatol ogy-info/glossary.htm.
- The University of Washington provides a dictionary of hundreds of technical/medical terms at eduserv.hscer.washington.edu/dermUW/lang.
- How to read a prescription: www.oag.state.med.us/ Consumer/ibt1.htm.
- Medical abbreviations: www.ucc.ie/info/net/acronyms/ index.html.

GENERAL ECZEMA AND MEDICINE INFORMATION

- DermNet has information on a variety of skin diseases, their causes, summaries of the disease, and investigations into future treatments. It also has links to academic institutions. The main Web site is www.dermnet.org.nz.
- The Food and Drug Administration offers a comprehensive catalog and descriptive profile of each new drug approved by the FDA in the past decade at www.centerwatch.com/drugs/druglist.htm.
- The Hardin Meta Directory (Hardin MD) provides links to top Internet sources for information about skin disease. It searches a number of databases, including the National Library of Medicine and Medline: www.lib.uiowa.edu/hardin/md/derm.html.
- The "Common Integument" chapter of *Gray's Anatomy* online has a variety of photos and illustrations of the skin that can be resized for optimal viewing: www.bartleby.com/107/234.html.
- There are two Web sites for the general public that explain how the immune system works: www.cellsalive.com/antibody.htm and the anatomy of the immune system, www.micro.msb.le.ac.uk/MBChB/2b.html.

SEARCH ENGINES

- MDChoice is a search tool that lets users enter a question and get back reviews, original research, or commentary. This can be used to pull up articles for the general public as well as specialists: www.mdchoice.com/medline.asp.
- The National Institutes of Arthritis and Musculoskeletal

and Skin Diseases is the branch of the NIH dealing specifically with skin disease, including eczema. It offers its own search engine with tips to refine searches: www.nih.gov/niams/niamssearchengine.htm.

CURRENT STANDARD OF CARE

Clinical guidelines are outlines defining standard treatments of diseases. The government-sponsored National Guideline Clearinghouse is at www.guideline.gov and can be searched by keyword (for instance, "eczema").

FUTURE RESEARCH

- Center Watch catalogs preclinical and clinical research on a number of diseases, including eczema. It organizes the information by topic and geographic locale of the facilities and providers conducting the research.
- www.centerwatch.com/patient/nih/nih_index.html.
- www.clinicaltrials.gov.
- For those in Canada: www.medistudy.com/clinical_trials/index.html.
- Medical breakthroughs can be accessed via www.ivanhoe.com/#reports, which updates and posts daily news in the health care field; you can also have them sent to your e-mail address.

SUPPORT GROUPS

- Support group sponsored by the American Academy of Dermatology: www.aad.org/foundations.html.

- University of Iowa College of Medicine's Dermatology Patient Support and Advocacy Groups: tray.dermatology.uiowa.edu/SuprtGrps.html.
- National Eczema Association for Science and Education: www.eczema-assn.org.
- The American Academy of Allergy Asthma and Immunology has useful links for eczema and related syndromes in the atopic triad: www.aaaai.org.

ADVOCACY

- www.congress.org is a directory of members of the Capitol, the Supreme Court, and the White House and state governors. Comments on members of Congress by different advocacy groups and associations can be found. You can determine a bill's status, send messages to member of Congress, and find local congressional representatives in your area.
- Families USA is a nonprofit organization dedicated to achieving high-quality and affordable health care for all Americans. Its Web site has information on Medicare, Medicaid, managed care, children's health, and what to do if you're uninsured. Their Web site is www.familiesusa.org.
- Health insurance is monitored by the Agency for Healthcare Research and Quality. The site discusses types of insurance (fee for service, helath maintenance organization, preferred provider organization; Medicare, Medicaid, hospital indemnity insurance, disability insurance, and long-term care insurance). They also have a checklist of things to consider when choosing insurance: www.ahcpr.gov/consumer/insurance.htm.
- The Employer Quality Partnership is sponsored by em-

ployers and is designed to educate employees regarding employer-based health plans. It is found at www.eqp.org

ALTERNATIVE MEDICINE

The National Center for Complementary and Alternative Medicine looks into current information on herbal therapies as well as consensus reports, clinical trial information, and future research. It has important links to federal resources. See www.nccam.nih.gov.

LABORATORY TESTS

Skin biopsy is described in step-by-step detail at the University of Utah's Web site: medstat.med.utah.edu/kw/derm/proced/punch.htm.

FUTURE READING

The *Merck Manual* online features chapter 174, "Skin Infections," describing how to recognize disorders: www.merck.com/pubs/mmanual_home/sec17/174.htm.

BOOKS

Common Skin Disorders. Ernst Epstein, W. B. Saunders Co., 2001.

20 Common Problems in Dermatology. Alan Fleischer, McGraw-Hill, 2002.

Atopic Dermatitis. Kristian Thestrup Pederson and Tim J. David, Dunitz Martin Ltd. Publication planned for March 2006 (ISBN 1841841447).

Pocket Guide to Eczema and Contact Dermatitis. Colin Holden and Lucy Ostlere, Blackwell Science, Inc., 2001.

The Official Patient's Sourcebook on Atopic Dematitis. James N. Parker and Phillip M. Parker, Icon Health Publications, 2002.

MEDICATIONS

- Medline site describes antihistamine medications and factors to be aware of when using them: www.nlm.nih.gov/medlineplus/druginfo/antihistaminessystemic202060.html.
- The FDA offers a comprehensive catalog and descriptive profile of each new drug approved by the FDA in the past decade: www.centerwatch.com/drugs/druglist.htm.

OCCUPATIONAL ECZEMA

- Occupational hazards for the skin can be found at the National Institute of Occupational Safety and Health's Web site: www.cdc.gov/niosh/ocderm.html#index.
- There is also a database of occupations in which allergic contact dermatitis is a hazard: www.haz-map.com/workers.htm.

COSMETICS AND SKIN CARE PRODUCTS

- The Cosmetic, Toiletry, and Fragrance Association evaluates personal care products such as makeup, skin protectants, soaps, and cleansers and publishes the results on www.ctfa.org.
- The FDA also publishes evaluations of cosmetics and the cosmetic industry at vm.cfsan.fda.gov/~dms/cos-toc.html.

- Ingredients of cosmetic preparations can be found at www.fda.gov/fdac/reprints/puffery.html.
- The National Library of Medicine offers information for consumers on cosmetics, labeling, fragrances, and hair and nail products. It also has a special health section for teenagers. See www.medlineplus.nlm.nih.gov/medlineplus/cosmetics.html.

ORGANIZATIONS

- Eczema Association of Australasia Inc.
  ABN 47 072 394 542
  P.O. Box 1784 DC, Cleveland QLD 4163, Australia
  Phone: 1300-300-182 or 07-3821-3297
  Information and Memberships: help@eczema.org.au
  Administration: itchy@eczema.org.au
- The newsletter provides a great deal of up-to-date information and publishes a useful online newsletter that keeps subscribers abreast of the latest developments in eczema treatment.
- newsletter@eczema.org.au
- Fujisawa Corporation publishes information on their product, Protopic (tacrolimus), a potent topical immunomodulator for the treatment of eczema. *The Fujisawa Handbook on Eczema for Kids* is available as a downloadable .pdf file and has lots of great tips for eczema in children. There's also a portal into a chat room for people with eczema to confidentially discuss their concerns with others who also suffer from the disease. See www.undermyskin.com.
- The Gateway to Asthma, Allergy, Intolerance Information on the Web is a clearinghouse for all things related to

atopic disorders, including asthma, allergic rhinitis, and atopic dermatitis: www.allallergy.net.

- The British Eczema Association is a nonprofit Web site that provides information about United Kingdom resources for eczema.
  National Eczema Society
  Hill House, Highgate Hill, London, N19 5NA
  Phone: 020-7281-3553
  Fax: 020-7281-6395
  E-mail: www.eczema.org
- National Eczema Association for Science and Education
  4460 Redwood Highway, Street 16-D
  San Rafael, California 94903-1953
  Phone: (415) 499-3474 / (800) 818-7546
  Fax: (415) 472-5345
  Web site: www.eczema-assn.org
  E-mail: info@nationaleczema.org
- The Eczema Mailing List allows people with eczema to share their experiences of living with and managing eczema. The list is also open to parents of children with eczema and people with a professional interest in eczema. It is not open to those with commercial interests or people wishing to advertise products or services. See website.lineone.net/~eczema/.
- The National Jewish Hospital in Denver Colorado specializes in atopic diseases: www.nationaljewish.org/diseases/dt18.html.
- Lung Line lets you talk directly to nurses about eczema Monday through Friday, from 8:00 a.m. to 4:30 p.m., mountain time. In addition to answering your questions, they can send you free educational materials and refer you to a specialist, if indicated.

Lung Line
National Jewish Medical and Research Center
1400 Jackson Street
Denver, Colorado 80206
Phone: (800) 222-LUNG (5864)
Outside the United States, call (303) 388-4461
E-mail: lungline@njc.org
Society of Pediatric Dermatology
Web site: www.pedsderm.net.

PRODUCTS FOR SENSITIVE SKIN

Cleansers

Albolene
Eucerin Cleansing Bar
Johnson's Baby Bar
Oilatum AD

Moisturizers

Aquaphor
Aveeno Lotion
Elta Crème, Eucerin Cream
Pond's Cold Cream
SBR Lipocream
Impruv
Theraplex Clear Lotion
Theraplex Emollient

Sunscreen

Neutrogena Sensitive Skin Sunblock
Clinique City Block Chemical Free

Shampoo: DHS Clear Shampoo

Conditioner: DHS Conditioning Rinse
Shaving Cream for Men: Neutrogena Razor Defense

Makeup

Lipstick: Adrien Arpel Powder Cream Lipstick
Adrien Arpel 2 Powdery Cream
Trish McEvoy Cream Powder

Blush

Dubarry Bloom Powder Cheek Tint
Elizabeth Arden Luxury Crème-to-Powder Blush

Loose Powder

Chanel Translucent
Laszlo Controlling Face Powder

Pressed Powder

Almay Matte Finish
Almay Oil Blotting Powder

Eyeliner

Chanel Smudge Eyeliner Pencil
Max Factor Eyebrow and Eyeliner Pencil

Mascara

Dior Thickening Lash Care
Sisley Botanical Mascara

Eye Shadow

Stagelight Matte Eye Powder

Index

Page numbers in *italics* refer to illustrations.

abdomen, 76, 202
abscesses, 70, 199, 216
Acarex, 96
Acarosan, 99
Ace bandages, 83
acidic soaps, 56
acids, 56
acne, 199
acute rashes, 49
additives, 60
adenoids, *30*
adolescents, teenagers, xxii, 165–67
advocacy, patient, *see* patient advocacy
age, 19, 49
agitation, 38
Agriculture Department, U.S. (USDA), 19
air cleaners, 92–94
air-conditioning, 92, 153
alcohol, 57, 81
alcoholic beverages, 43, 62, 149, 165
alkaline chemicals, 108
alkaline soaps, 56
alkylbenzene sulfonates, 109
alkylolamides, 109
alkylpolyglycosides, 109
allantoinate, 81
allergens, 34, 44, 46, 58, 74, 147, 186, 199
allergic contact dermatitis, 67, 199
allergic rhinitis, xxii, 14, *15,* 16, 27, 155, 194, 200, 205
allergic shiners, 10
allergies, 34, 59, 61, 76, 199, 207
Allergy Control Solution, 99
all-natural ingredients, 59
aloe vera, 59, 123
alopecia (hair loss), 12–13
alpha-hydroxy acid, 80
alpha-olefin sulfonates, 109
alternative medicine, 168
aluminum chloride, 81
aluminum hydroxide, 81
aluminum sulfate, 81

index

American Academy of Dermatology, 150
Americans with Disabilities Act, 110
amino acids, 59
anaphylaxis, anaphylactic shock, 70, 212
anesthetic gels, 66
anger, 77, 127, 169–70
antibiotics, 25, 62, 144, 185
antibodies, 32, 200
antifoaming agents, 60
antifungals, 186
antihistamines, 65, 69, 74, 123, 144, 147, 154, 165, 183, 187, 219
antimicrobial medication, 185–86
antimite solutions, 99
antiperspirants, deodorants, 81
antiseptics, 67, 72, 186
antisocial behavior, 149
anus, 122
armpits, underarms, 83, 202
arms, 76
aromatherapy, 189–90
artificial colors, 57, 79
artificial nails, 81
Aspercreme, 64
aspirin, 45, 64, 66
assertiveness training, 126
asteatotic eczema, 200
asthma, xxii, 4, 14–15, *15,* 16, 27, 155, 194, 200, 205
atopic, 200
atopic dermatitis, xxi, 200
  see also eczema
atopic triad, 14, *15,* 16, 200, 205
atopy, 200
atrophy, 200
attorneys, 112
auto exhaust, 85
autoimmune disease, 207
Aveeno, 56, 123
Aveeno for Men, 81

Bacitracin, 67
bacteria, 8, 23, 25, 82, 107
balneotherapy, 197, 200
bandaging, 72–73, 144, 153, 155
Band-Aids, 68, 73
barrier, skin, *24, 26, 28,* 29, 34, *36,* 37, 44, 46, 48, 109, 155, 184, 201, 205, 206, 208
  artificial, 195
  faulty function of, xxi, 42, 196
basement, 90
basement membrane, 23–25
basophils, 201, 202, 204
bathing, baths, 55–57, 152, 201
  of infants, 141–42
bath oils, 56
B cells, 200, 202, 203, 204, 205, 207
bed bugs, 100
bedding, 96–98
bedtime, 152–55
behavioral therapy, 172
Benadryl, 65, 69, 147
benzalkonium chloride (Zephiran), 72
benzene, 100, 101
benzocaine, 123
benzoyl benzoate, 99
benzoyl peroxide, 80
benzyl alcohol, 60
Betadine (iodine), 67
betaine, 109
biofeedback, 186
biofilm, 25
biologics, 196–97
biopsy, skin, 201
bioresonance therapy, 190
birth defects, 119, 120
blepharitis, 202
blisters, 9, 32, 54, 70, 71
blood vessels, 22, 24, 25, 30, 31, 32, 42, 43, 91, 128–29, 131
body lice, 211
boils, 70
bone, 12
bone marrow, *30,* 200, 201, 202, 210
brain, 12, 37, 43, 45, 47, 48, 164
breast-feeding, 120, 193
breasts, 76, 202
bulla, bullae, 202

caffeine, 43, 76, 175
calamine lotion, 66, 67, 68, 69
camphor, 66, 69, 123

index

cancer, skin, 122, 189, 210, 212, 214, 218
candida, 71, 202
Capsaicin, 186
carbon monoxide, 101
carbuncle, 216
career choice, 103–6
carpets, 91, 98
cars, 84
cataracts, 212, 214
cells:
  antigen-presenting, 29, 30
  B, 200, 202, 203, 204, 205, 207
  epidermal, 29, *36*
  immune, 25, 29, 30, *30,* 31, 32, 34, 43
  Langerhans, 202, 204, 205, 208, 218
  mast, 29, 202, 204, 210
  nerve, 47, 210
  skin, 47
  T, *33,* 188, 189, 202, 203, 204, 205, 217
  Th1, *33,* 186, 217
  Th2, *33,* 186, 217
cell surface receptors, 31
cellulitis, 202, 216
ceramide, 58
cerebral cortex, 38
cetyl alcohol, 60
cetyl palmitate, 60
C fibers, 38
chalk dust, 149
chicken pox, 156
childhood eczema, 139–60, 161–76
  emotional repercussions of, 162–64
  environment and, 140
  first aid for, 144–45
  healthy habits and, 145
  psychological issues in, 161–76
  remedies for itching in, 146–47
  and school issues, 149–50
  use of rewards in, 148, 155, 170
childhood illnesses, 155–56
chills, 144
Chinese medicine, 183
chlorine (Clorox), 55, 67, 96
chlorobutanol, 60
chlorpheniramine, 65
Chlor-Trimeton, 65
chromosomes, 27, 28
chronic rashes, 49
cigarettes, 73, 94, 149, 153, 165
cimetidine, 65
circadian cycles, 37
Claritin, 65
clay, 149
cleanliness, xxii, 34, 141
climate, 115
Clorox (chlorine), 55, 67, 96
clothing, 78–80
Coban, 155
Cochrane Review, 180
cockroach droppings, 95
code molecules, 28
cold, 42–43
cold compresses, 64, 67
cold hands, 13
cold sores, 202–3
  see also herpes simplex virus
collagen, *24,* 25, 59
Colloidin, 108
complexion, 4
compresses, lukewarm, 68
conception, 118
conjunctiva, 11
contact dermatitis, 203
copayment, 111
Corbusier, Le (Charles Édouard Jeanneret), 88
cornified envelope, 23
cornstarch, 64
corticosteroid, 203
cortisol levels, 37
cosmetics, 58, 80
counseling, 133
coworkers, 110
cracking, *see* fissuring
cradle cap, 203, 216
creams, 58, 61, 146, 152, 155, 156, 183
crust, crusting, 4, 8, 54, 67, 70, 144–45
crying, 154–55
cuticles, 9
cuts, 54, 72–73, 83, 116, 152
cyclomethicone, 59

cyclosporine (Neoral), 118, 119, 181
cysts (milia), 14
cytokines, *33,* 43, 47, 196, 197, 203
cytokine signatures, *33*

Dacron, 98
dampness, 86, 89, 95
see also humidity
dander, 73, 95, 96, 98, 99, 105, 153
dandruff, 152, 216
defensins, 197
Denny-Morgan folds, 11
depression, 125, 130–31, 166–67
clinical, 130
reactive, 130
dermal-epidermal junction, 31
dermatitis, 204
dermatologists, 17, 19, 61, 68, 74, 158, 160
dermatophytosis, 204
dermis, 22, 23, *24,* 25, *26,* 29, 30, 31, 200, 201, 204, 206, 207, 210
detergents, 109, 190
diaper rash, 142
diary, 148
diets, 75
elimination, 190
infant and maternal, 193–94
dimethicone, 59
discharge, 71
discoid (nummular) eczema, 204, 211
discoloration, 71, 145
dispersing agents, 60
DNA, 28
doctor-patient relationship, 17–21
dolphins, 188
dorsal root ganglia (DRG), 38
double helix, 28
Dove soap, 56–57
doxepin (Zonalon) cream, 66, 147
DRG (dorsal root ganglia), 38
drugs, illegal, 149, 166
dry cleaning, 79
dry skin, dryness, 54, 55, 121, 156
dust, 73, 94, 98, 153
dust mites, 62, 86, 90, 91, 94, 95–100, 153
allergen injections for, 186
desensitization to, 184
elimination of, 184–85
dyphenhydramine, 65

Eames, Charles and Ray, 88
eczema, 204
asteatotic, 200
childhood, 139–60, 161–76
diagnosing of, 3–16
discoid (nummular), 204, 211
disorders related to, 14–16
genetic basis of, 27–34
hand, 102–9, 206
herpeticum, 203
nipple, 210
relapsing, 74
related disorders, *see specific disorders*
signs associated with, 12–14
symptoms of, 4–12
systematic indicators of, 11–12
weeping, 67
whole-body, *28*
elastin, *24,* 59
elbows, 6, 49, 143
Elidel (pimecrolimus), 122, 159, 189
emollients, 60, 66, 83, 118, 119, 120, 121, 147, 152, 156, 158, 185, 201, 205, 207
emotional distress, 124–26
emotions:
family and, 134–36
and flares, 124–26
management of, 124–36
negative, 126–31
positive, 131–34
emulsifying agents, 60
endorphins, 43, 176
environmental stimuli, *28*
enzymes, 59, 190
eosinophils, 202, 204, 205
epidermis, 22, 23–25, *24, 26,* 29, 30, 31, 32, 200, 201, 205, 206, 207, 208, 218
epinephrine, self-injectable, 70
erysipelas, 216
erythema, 205
erythroderma, 205
erythromycin, 45

estrogen, 203
ethoxylated fatty acid glycerides, 109
ethoxylated fatty alcohols, 109
ethylenediamine, 60
excoriation (scratch marks), 8
exercise, 77, 78
eyebrows, 13
eyelids, 6, 10–11, 14, 82, 202
eyes, 3, 6, 10–11, 82

fabrics, 78, 191
face, 10, 49, 141, 143, 156
facial products, 42
factories, 85
family relationships, 134–36
  communication in, 134–35
  keeping peace in, 170–71
  parent-child, 135, 167–71, 175–76
  sibling jealousy in, 172–74
  with teenagers, 165–66
fatigue, 12, 38
fatty acids, 184, 196
fatty alcohol ether sulfates, 109
fatty tissue, 25
FDA (Food and Drug Administration), 112, 118
fear, 128
feet, 83
feminine hygiene products, 123
fever, 32, 69, 144
fever blister, 205
fiberglass, 42, 44, 89–90, 98
fibroblasts, 204
"fight or flight" response, 43, 203
fingernails, 9, 71, 81–82, 149
fingers, 71, 82, 202
fissuring, 9, 54, 66–67, 68, 71, 121, 143, 206
flares, 73–74
  emotions and, 124–26
flat wart, 206
fleas, 100
flooring, 91
folliculitis, 70, 206, 216
Food and Drug Administration (FDA), 112, 118
food coloring, 63
food handling, 80
formaldehyde, 100, 101, 123
frustration, 77
fungus, fungal infection, 10, 64, 70, 82, 115, 121, 122, 145, 149, 204, 206, 211, 212, 215
furuncle, 216

generic medications, 172
genes, *28,* 199
gene therapy, 198
genetics, xxi, 27–34, 140, 192
genital area, 70, 76, 120, 121–23
geographic tongue (lingual erythema migrans), 10
germs, 34, 146
gloves, 79–80, 106–7, 143, 147
Gloves in a Bottle, 107, 108, 195
glucose, 64
glue, 149
glycerin, 60
glyceryl monostearate, 60
glycolic acid, 81
Gold Bond Medicated Powder, 64, 66
gooseflesh (keratosis pilaris), 13
groin, 121
guilt, 167–68
guinea pigs, 84
gum tragacanth, 60

hair follicles, 22, *24,* 199
hair loss (alopecia), 12–13
hand eczema, 102–9, 206
hands, 79, 102–9
  washing of, 80, 109, 146
hayfever, *see* allergic rhinitis
head lice, 211
health care management, 17–21
heart, 12
heat, 42–43, 44, 48, 62, 107, 142, 153
hemorrhoids, 122
HEPA (high-efficiency particulate air) filter, 92
herbal medicine, Chinese, 183
herb tea, 183
herpes simplex virus, 70, 71, 156–57, 202, 206, 219

Hertoghe's sign, 13
hexachlorophene, 60
high-efficiency particulate air (HEPA) filter, 92
Hindle, Tim, 175
histamine, 43, 154, 201, 206, 210
hives, 218
Hollofil, 98
home, location of, 85–86
home construction materials, 89–91
home environment, 85–101
  exterior, 85–91
  interior, 91–101
home furnishings, 98–100
home heating, 92
hospitalization, 186
housekeeping, 103
houseplants, 100–101
  see also plants
Human Genome Project, 27, 192
human papillomavirus, 206, 207, 219
humectant, 207
humidifiers, 94
humidity, 42, 44, 73, 94
  see also dampness
hydrocarbons, 183
hydrocortisone, 66, 69, 122
hydrogen peroxide, 72
hyperkeratosis (scale), 4, 6
hyperlinearity, 14
hypersensitivity, 207
hypertension, 181
hypnosis, 43, 172
hypnotherapy, 186
hypoallergenic, 59
hypotension, 12

ice, 64, 69
ichthyosis, 207
idleness, 63
IgE (immunoglobulin E), 37, 188, 207
imagery, 164–65
immune barrier, *26*
immune cells, 25, 29, 30, *30,* 31, 32, 34, 43, 204
immune response, xxi, 34, 37, 47, 126, 189, 197, 201, 210
immune system, xxii, 15, *28,* 29–34, *33, 36,* 37, 44, 119, 125, 126, 128, 140, 145, 189, 191, 199, 201, 202, 203, 207, 208, 209, 215, 218
immunoglobulin, 207–8
immunoglobulin E (IgE), 37, 188, 207
immunomodulator, 181
impetigo, 208, 216
Impruv, 108
infant care, 103
infants, infancy, xxii, 140–42, 193–94
infections, 8, 9, 11, *36,* 47, 66–73, 74, 82, 144, 145, 146, 156–57, 185
inflammation, 4, 5, 29, 31, 32–34, 36, 37, 208
insect bites, 42, 69–70
insect control, natural, 87
insecticides, 87
insects, 87–88, 90, 93
insulation materials, 89–90
insurance companies, 19, 20
insurance coverage, 110–12, 172, 174–75
intercourse, 121
interferon, *33*
interferon gamma injections, 186–87
Internet, 113, 116, 160
iodine (Betadine), 67
ion generators, 93, 94
iron oxide, 108
irritability, 38
irritants, xxi, *36,* 37, 44, 46, 73, 74, 208
  mechanical, 42
  from within, 43
isethionates, 109
isolation, 166, 169
isopropyl alcohol, 109
isopropyl myristate, 60
itching, xxii, 3, 4, 9, 23, 31, 32, 36–46, 68, 71, 121, 122, 208
  causes of, 61–63
  in children, 146–49, 164–65
  genital, 123
  in infants, 140–42
  irritants and, 38–44
  mind and, 43
  nighttime, 37–38, 56, 62
  nonchemical relief of, 63–65

pain vs., 36–37, 47–48
physiology of, 38
rating scale for, 35
research on, 195
soothing of, 63–66
triggers for, 38–44, 62–63
types of, 44–46
itch nerve receptors, 46
itch-scratch-itch cycle, 45, 142
itch-scratch-rash cycle, 35–49, 61–62
itch triggers, 38–44, 62–63
It's About Time! (Sapadin), 175

Jeanneret, Charles Édouard (Le Corbusier), 88
joints, 6
jojoba oil, 59

keloids, 208
keratinocytes, 23, 205, 207, 208
keratoconus, 11
keratosis pilaris (gooseflesh), 13
Kerlix, 155
kidney failure, 181
kidneys, 12
knees, 6, 49, 143

landscaping, 86–87
Langerhans cells, 202, 204, 205, 208, 218
latex, 123
laughter, 132, 176
laundry products, 79
leather, 149
legs, 76
levamisole, 191
lice, 211
lichenification, 4, 7, 8, 121, 209
lichen simplex chronicus, 209
lidocaine, 66
lingual erythema migrans (geographic tongue), 10
lipids, 23, *26,* 196, 204, 209
lips, 70, 83, 156
liver, 12
loratadine, 65
lotions, 58, 61, 77, 116
lubricants, 60
lukewarm compresses, 68
lymph, 209
lymphadenopathy (enlarged lymph glands), 11, 69
lymphatic channels, *24,* 209, 210
lymphatic vessels, *30,* 31
lymph glands, enlarged (lymphadenopathy), 11, 69
lymph nodes, 3, 11, *24,* 30, *30,* 31, 32, 69, 202, 208, 209
lymphocyte, 210

maceration, 202
macule, 210
magainins, 23
magnesium oxide, 81
makeup, 42, 149
malaise, 144
male fertility, 119
malnutrition, 12
Manage Your Time (Hindle), 175
marigolds, 87
massage, 142, 155, 185, 190
mast cells, 29, 202, 204, 210
materials safety data sheet (MSDS), 106
media, 114–15, 160
medical alert bracelet, 70
medical history, 19
medications, 62, 65, 66, 74, 77
meditation, 43, 77, 152
melanin, 7, 210
melanocytes, 7, 205, 210, 219
menstruation, 117–18
menthol, 66, 69, 123
metallic salts, 81
methotrexate (MTX), 118–19
methylcellulose, 60
methylparabin, 60
Mies van der Rohe, Ludwig, 88
milia (cysts), 14
mineralocorticoids, 203
moisturizers, 55, 57–58, 68, 116, 120, 143, 148, 158
moisturizing, 55, 57–61
mold, 86, 89, 90, 94, 95–96, 98, 210
molluscum contagiosum, 157, 210, 219

moods, 131–32
Mosquito Deleto, 87
Mosquito Magnet, 87
motor cortex, 38
motor nerves, 25
mouth, 6, 13, 71
MSDS (materials safety data sheet), 106
MTX (methotrexate), 118–19
mud baths, 117
mupirocin, 185
muscles, 12, *24*
music, 175
mycosis fungoides, 210

nail trimming, 144, 147
Nalgene, 116
NASA, 100
nasturtiums, 87
National Eczema Association for Science and Education (NEASE), 115, 132, 139, 150, 172
neck, 6, 49, 76
neomycin, 67
Neoral (cyclosporine), 118, 119, 181
Neosporin, 67
nerve cells (neurons), 47, 210
nerve endings, 23, 25, 48, 205
nerves, 22, *24,* 31, 32, 38, 43, 45, 210
neurodermatitis, 125
neurogenic itch, 45
nickel dermatitis, 199, 210
nighttime itching, 56, 62, 76
nipple eczema, 210
nipples, 6, 83, 120
nitrazepan, 191
Nivea, 58
nodules, 210
nonsedating antihistamines, 65
nose, 81
nucleic acids, 59
nummular (discoid) eczema, 204, 211
nurses, 187

oatmeal baths, xxii, 56, 57, 146
occlusion (wraps), 120
Occupational Safety and Health Administration (OSHA), 105
oil glands, 22
ointments, 58, 61, 153
Olay Sensitive Skin, 57
onychomychosis, 211
oolong tea, 188
oozing, 54, 66, 67, 68
opium-based pain medications, 45, 62
optical brighteners, 79
organic, 59
organic oils, 108
organic solvents, 108
oxyquinolone sulfate, 60
ozone, 93

PAF (platelet activating factor) antagonist, 187
Paget's disease, 210
pain, 47, 71
pallor, 13
palms, 6, 14
papillae, 25
papillomavirus, *see* human papillomavirus
papule, 211
parabens, 60
parachlorometaxylenol, 60
parasites, 37, 44
parasitosis, 211
parents:
  psychological effects on, 167–72
  tips for, 159–60
particulate pollution, 92
patch testing, 211
patient advocacy, 112–15, 150
  legislators and, 114
  media and, 114
patient-centered care, 17
pediculus humanus capitis (head lice), 211
pediculus humanus corporis (body lice), 211
Pei, I. M., 88
penis, 121, 122
peptides, 197
perfumes, 57, 79, 149
perioral dermatitis, 211
permanent press fabrics, 123
perspiration, *see* sweat, sweating
petroleum jelly, 58, 72, 73, 141, 143, 147

pets, 44, 83–84, 99, 100, 153
Peyer's patches, *30*
pH, 56–57
phantom limb sensation, 45
phototherapy, 211–12
phthirus pubis, 211
physical barrier, *26*
pimecrolimus (Elidel), 122, 159, 189
pinworms, 122
pityriasis alba, 212
pityriasis versicolor, 212
plants, 86–87
  see also houseplants
plants, beneficial, 101
plaque, 212
plastic, 149
platelet-activating factor (PAF) antagonist, 187
platelets, 202
poison ivy dermatitis, 212–13
pollens, 44, 73, 84, 86, 89, 92, 93, 94, 95, 98
pollutants, 86
polyester, 78
polyethylene glycol, 60
polymers, *26*
polymyxin B, 67
Polysporin, 67
pompholyx, 213
pores, 25
potassium permanganate, 67
povidone-iodine (Betadine), 72
poxvirus, 157, 210
pramoxine, 123
pregnancy, 62, 119–20, 194
preservatives, 60
prick testing, 213
primary care doctor, 19
probiotics, 194
propylparabin, 60
proteins, 23, *26,* 29, 59
Proteque, 108
Protopic (tacrolimus), 122, 159
prurigo nodularis, 213
pruritoceptive itch, 44, 45
pruritus, 213
Psoralen, 122, 214
Psoralen ultraviolet A (PUVA), 122, 212, 214
psoriasis, 122, 200, 213
psychogenic itch, 45–46
psychological impact, 161–76
psychological therapy, 174–75, 181
psychotherapy, 172
pubic lice, 211
pubis, 121
pus, 69, 199
pustules, 54, 70, 214
PUVA (Psoralen ultraviolet A) 122, 212, 214

quarternary ammonium compounds, 60

radioallergosorbent test (RAST), 215
ranitidine (Zantac), 187
rashes, xxi, xxii, 3, 4, 5, 8, 9, 12, 49, 214
RAST (radioallergosorbent test), 215
redness, 54, 71, 120, 121, 122, 144
refrigeration, 147
relaxation, 78, 144, 152, 181
religion, 176
retinol, 81
rhinitis, allergic, *see* allergic rhinitis
ringworm, 214
RNA, 29, 59
Roach Motel, 87
rubber, 149
Rutter scale of psychological disturbance, 163

salicylic acid, 81, 121
saline compress, 68
salons, spas, 82
salt baths, 187, 197
salt water, 117
saltwater treatments, 117
Sapadin, Linda, 175
scab, 8
scabies, 122, 215
scaling (hyperkeratosis), 4, 6, 71, 121, 122
scalp, 13, 121, 141, 143, 152
school issues, 149–50, 166–67
scrapes, *see* cuts

scratching, xxii, 4, *36,* 46–49, 54, 74, 142–43, 144, 148, 154–55, 215
scratch marks (excoriation), 4, 8, 144, 152
scrotum, 122
seaweed wraps, 117
sebaceous glands, 10, *24,* 25, 216
seborrheic dermatitis, 216
sebum, *24*
secondary alkane sufonates, 109
sedating antihistamines, 65
sedation, 76
self-blame, 127
self-care routine, *see* skin care routine, daily
self-loathing, 127
sensory cortex, 38
sensory nerves, 25
serum, 8, 32
"seven-year itch," 215
sex, 19
sexual health, 117–23
shampooing, 56
shock, 12
showering, 56
siblings, 172–74
silicone, 59
siloxane, 59
skin:
  dry, 4, 6, 10
  leaky, 9
  physiology of, 22–26
  signs and symptoms, 4–10
skin care products, 172
  in workplace, 108–9
skin care routine, daily, 53–74
  bathing in, 55–57
  managing flares in, 73–74
  managing infection in, 66–73
  moisturizing in, 57–61
  scheduling for, 54
  skin inspection in, 54
skin color, altered, 7
skin folds, 64, 71, 202
sleep, 76, 145, 151–55
sleep deprivation, 37–38, 152
smallpox, 155
smoking, *see* cigarettes
soaps, 55, 56–57, 109, 116
Society for Pediatric Dermatology, 150
sodium lauryl sulfate, 60
soles, 6
spa, 117
spinal cord, 38
spirituality, 176
spleen, *30,* 216
sports, 82–83
staphylococcal bacteria, 23
staphylococcal infection, 23, 70, 208, 216
staphylococcal-scalded skin syndrome, 70
Staphylococcus aureus, 70, 72, 156, 185, 216
stasis dermatitis, 216
State Department, U.S., 115
stearic acid, 60
stearyl alcohol, 60
steroids, 157–59
  anabolic, 157, 203
  creams, 66, 74, 121, 156, 157–58
  ointments, 158
  oral, 120, 156
  topical, 118, 119, 122, 181–82
stimulants, 166
stratum corneum, 42, 195
streptococcal infections, 216
Streptococcus pyogenes, 216
stress, 44, 46, 62, 73, 74, 77–78, 103, 128, 140, 145, 148, 152, 167–69
  financial, 171–72
  psychological, 124–31, 161–76
  reduction in the home, 175–76
stress hormones, 43, 128
subacute rashes, 49
subcutaneous fat layer, 22
subcutis, 22, *24,* 25, *26,* 206, 217
Substance P, 48
suicide, xxii, 38
sulfosuccinates, 109
sun, 117
sunburn, 218
sunscreen, 83, 108, 120
suplatast tosilate, 188
supplements, dietary, 184
support groups, support systems, 77, 132, 181
suspending agents, 60

sweat, sweating, 42, 62, 82, 142
sweat glands, 22, *24,* 25
swimmers, swimming, 83
synthetic ingredients, 59

tacrolimus (Protopic), 122, 188
Tagamet, 65
tannic acid, 99
tar, 117, 121, 183
T cells, *33,* 188, 189, 202, 203, 204, 205, 217
temperature, ambient, 42–43, 44, 73, 82, 91
temperature, body, 34, 43, 78
testosterone, 203
Th1, *33,* 186, 217
Th2, *33,* 186, 217
thalamus, 38
therapy, psychological, 174–75, 181
Theraseal, 108
thickening, *see* lichenification
thighs, 83, 121
thymic extracts, 188
thymopentin, 188
thymus, *30,* 217
tinea, 215, 217
titanium, 83
titanium oxide, 108
TL101 lamp, 182
toddlers, 142–43
toes, 71, 202
toll receptors, 197
tongue, geographic (lingual erythema migrans), 10
tonsils, *30*
topical immunomodulators (TIMs), 122, 159, 188, 196
tranquilizers, 166
transfer factor, 189
traveling, 115–17
travel insurance, 116
travel kit, child's, 151
treatments, 17–21, 179–91
  first aid, 144–45
  for infants, 139–42
  for older children, 143–44
  positive mental state and, 131–34
  preventive, 193–95
  questions about, 20–21
  for toddlers, 142–43
trees, allergenic, 88
TriCeram cream, 58
triethanolamine, 81
"twilight sleep," 76

ulcers, 218
ultraviolet light, 218
ultraviolet radiation, 218
undergarments, 123
upholstery, 99
upper respiratory infection, 62
urushiol, 213
uticaria, 218–19
UVA (ultraviolet A), 182, 200, 212
UVB (ultraviolet B), 118, 120, 182, 212
UVC (ultra violet C), 182, 212
UV (ultraviolet) light, 121, 122, 182, 211–12
UV (ultraviolet) radiation, 122, 218

vaccines, 194–95
vacuum cleaning, 94–95
vaginal area, 71
varicose veins, 216
Vaseline Intensive Care Lotion, 58
vasodilatory foods, 62
verucca, 219
vesicles, 9, 219
Vicks VapoRub, 66
vinegar, 79
vinegar soak, 68
viral infections, 219
viruses, 156
vitamin B_2, 184
vitamin B_3, 196
vitamin E, 59, 184, 196
vitiligo, 7, 219
volatile organic compounds (VOCs), 79, 89, 98
vulva, 121

wall coverings, 98
warts, 157, 206, 219
water, 82

water-soluble compounds, 108
weeping eczema, 67, 158
weight, 76
weight loss, 12
wheals, 219
window dressings, 98
window filters, 93, 153
Wolverton, Bill, 100
Wood's lamp, 7
wool, 42, 62, 78, 98, 142, 149, 152
workplace, 78, 102–10, 169
  skin care products in, 108–9
wounds, 54, 72–73, 116
Wright, Frank Lloyd, 88

Xolair, 197

yeast, 121, 122, 202, 219
yoga, 78

Zantac (ranitidine), 187
Zeasorb AF powder, 107
Zephiran (benzalkonium chloride), 72
zinc, 83
zinc deficiency, 219
zinc oxide, 81, 108
zirconium chlorohydrate, 81
Zonalon (doxepin) cream, 66, 147

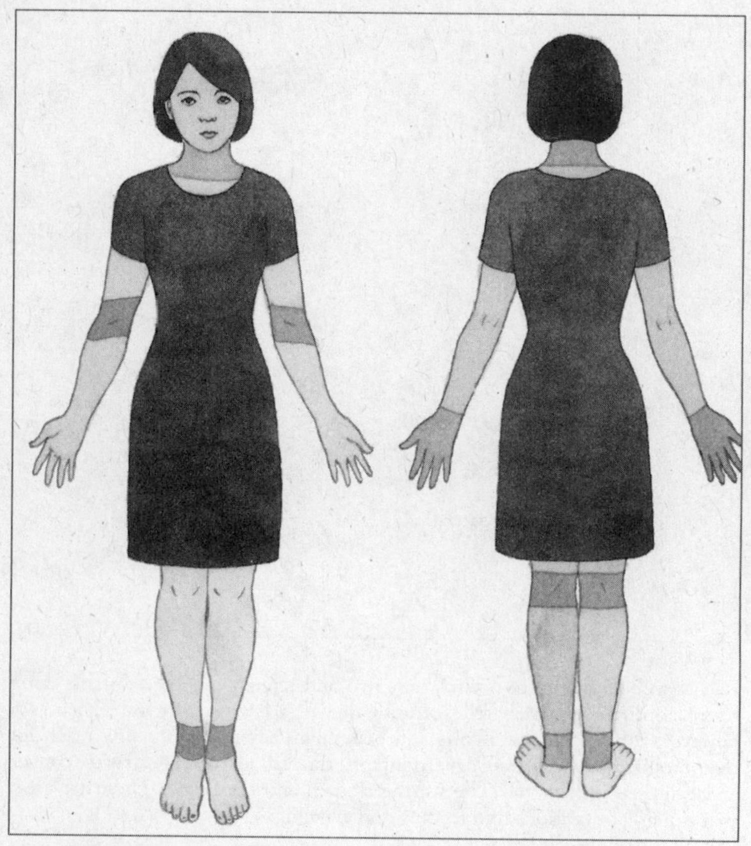

In children and adults, the rash tends to appear where itching is most severe. Commonly itching localizes in the skin folds. These trap sweat, irritants, and allergens. The barrier here is more likely to be disrupted from repeated bending and straightening and from friction against clothing and jewelry. Another common area in adults is the hands. Rashes on hands are common in adults and children who are exposed to chemicals or frequent handwashing.

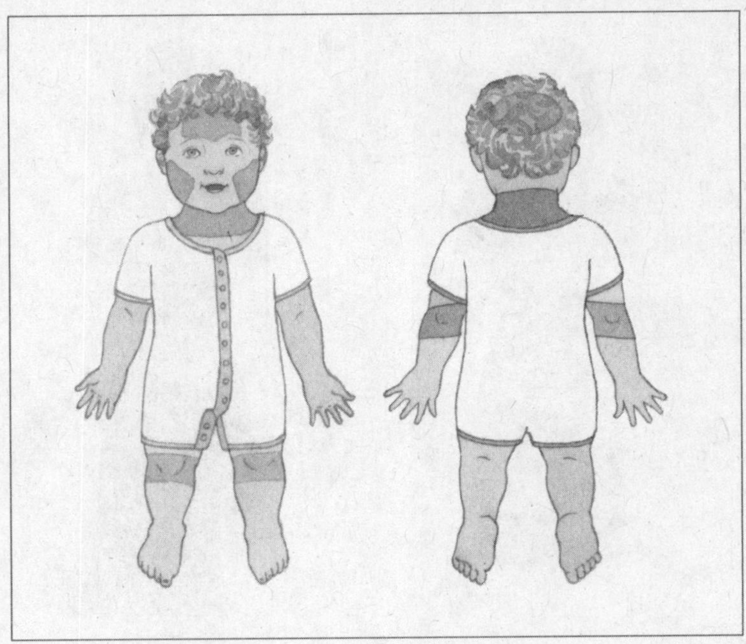

Rashes in babies tend to occur where itch and scratch converge. Infants don't have coordinated scratch reflexes until they're a few months old. They can, however, rub up against pillows and bedding. They also frequently reach for their mouth at a very young age. In infants, the rash tends to localize on convex and extensor surfaces: the cheeks, the elbows, and the knees. These are areas that experience friction from feeding and crawling.